PANCREATITIS DIET COOKBOOK FOR SENIORS

Nutritious and Easy Recipes to Support Digestive Health, Enhance Well-Being, and Promote a Comfortable Lifestyle

Kingsley Klopp

To show our appreciation for your purchase, we're delighted to offer you these special bonuses as a heartfelt thank you.

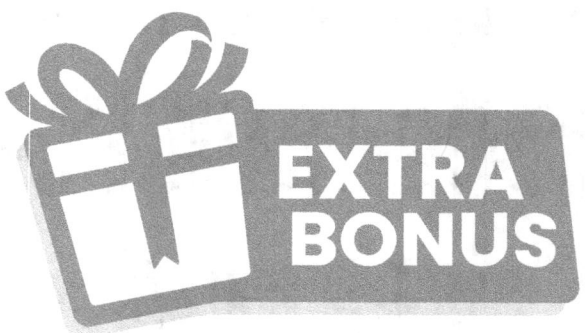

1. **A Food Tracker Journal**
2. **Downloadable E-BOOK featuring full-color images of finished recipes**

Copyright © 2024 All rights reserved.

No part of this book may be reproduced or transmitted in any form or by any means, electronic or mechanical, including photocopying, recording, or by any information storage and retrieval system, without written permission from the author. The scanning, uploading, and distribution of this book via the internet or via any other means without the permission of the author is illegal and punishable by law. The author has made every effort to ensure the accuracy of the information contained in this book. However, the author cannot be held responsible for any errors or omissions.

Table of Contents

Introduction..7

Chapter 1: Navigating Dietary Needs for Seniors
- Nutritional Needs for Seniors..9
- Common Dietary Challenges..11
- Tips for Maintaining a Healthy Diet..14

Chapter 2: Understanding Pancreatitis
- Types of Pancreatitis: Acute vs. Chronic..17
- Symptoms and Diagnosis..19
- Impact of Pancreatitis on Digestion..22

Chapter 3: Dietary Guidelines for Pancreatitis
- Foods to Avoid..24
- Foods to Include...27
- Reading Food Labels...30

Breakfast Recipes
Banana Oatmeal Porridge..33
Smoothie Bowl..34
Egg White Scramble...35
Avocado Toast on Whole Grain Bread..36
Peaches and Cream Smoothie..37
Carrot and Ginger Juice..38
Papaya Salad...39
Oat Bran Muffins..40
Buckwheat Pancakes..41
Vegetable Soup...42
Barley Porridge...43
Cucumber Tomato Sandwich...44
Chia Seed Pudding...45
Vegetable Omelette..46
Berry Fruit Salad...47

Pumpkin Soup..48
Mango Smoothie...49
Sautéed Vegetables...50
Almond Milk Porridge..51
Spelt Toast with Banana..52
Boiled Potatoes with Dill...53
Buckwheat Crepes..54
Rice and Pea Salad...55

Poultry Recipes
Herb-Roasted Turkey Breast...56
Chicken and Vegetable Soup..57
Ginger Chicken Stir-Fry...58
Lemon Garlic Chicken...59
Turkey Meatballs..60
Chicken Congee..61
Poached Chicken Salad..62
Smoked Turkey Wrap..63
Balsamic Chicken...64
Turkey and Rice Pilaf..65
Chicken Vegetable Kabobs...66
Orange-Glazed Chicken..67
Turkey Lettuce Cups...68
Chicken and Spinach Stew...69
Turkey Quinoa Stuffed Peppers..70
Chicken Cauliflower Fried Rice..71
Chicken Broth with Parsley..72
Turkey and Sweet Potato Skillet..73
Chicken Piccata..74
Chicken Ratatouille..75
Grilled Chicken with Peach Salsa..76
Chicken and Asparagus Lemon Stir Fry..77
Minty Turkey Patties..78
Chicken Pepperoni Marinara..79
Sage Turkey Loaf..80
Chicken and Mushroom Casserole..81
Grilled Turkey and Pineapple...82
Chicken and Broccoli Alfredo...83
Chicken Fajitas...84
Turkey and Parsnip Mash...85

Fish and Seafood Recipes
Grilled Salmon with Dill...86

Poached Cod..87
Baked Tilapia with Lemon Pepper...88
Shrimp and Vegetable Stir-Fry...89
Steamed Mussels with Garlic and Herbs..90
Crab Salad with Cucumber...91
Fish Soup with Tomatoes..92
Baked Trout with Rosemary...93
Grilled Shrimp Skewers...94
Scallops with Ginger and Soy...95
Flounder in Parchment..96
Lobster Steamed with Herbs..97
Fish Tacos with Cabbage Slaw...98
Sole Meunière...99
Squid Salad with Lime and Cilantro..100
Prawn Cocktail with Avocado...101
Baked Haddock with Tomatoes..102
Seared Tuna with Sesame Seeds..103
Broiled Scallops with Paprika...104
Fish Fillet with Parsley Sauce...105
Oysters on the Half Shell with Mignonette Sauce..................................106
Marinated Anchovies with Garlic and Vinegar.......................................107
Halibut Steaks with Herb Marinade..108
Stuffed Squid with Herbed Rice...109
Sardines Grilled with Lemon..110
Panko-Crusted Tilapia..111
Mackerel in Tomato Sauce..112
Peppered Mackerel on Rye...113
Grilled Eel with Teriyaki Sauce..114
Linguine with Clams..115
Monkfish with Saffron Broth..116

Soup & Stew Recipes
Carrot and Ginger Soup...117
Lentil and Spinach Soup..118
Chickpea and Vegetable Stew..119
Split Pea Soup...120
Pumpkin Soup...121
Bean and Barley Soup..122
Cabbage Soup..123
Vegetable Minestrone..124
Sweet Potato and Lentil Soup..125
Mushroom and Leek Soup..126

Zucchini and Basil Soup..127
White Bean and Kale Soup...128
Black Bean Soup..129
Broccoli and Potato Soup...130
Turmeric and Cauliflower Soup..131
Italian Vegetable Stew..132
Potato and Green Bean Soup..133
Chard and White Bean Soup...134

8-WEEK MEAL PLAN...135

Important Note

We are delighted to guide you through a collection of carefully curated recipes designed to support your health and well-being while living with pancreatitis. Before you embark on this culinary journey, we'd like to share a few important notes to ensure your experience is both safe and enjoyable.

Each individual's dietary needs are unique, especially when managing a condition as specific as pancreatitis. While the recipes in this cookbook are crafted with general guidelines for pancreatitis in mind, we recognize that what works well for one person may not be suitable for another. Therefore, we encourage you to listen to your body and adjust the recipes as needed to better align with your personal dietary requirements.

It's crucial to remember that this cookbook is intended to complement, not replace, professional medical advice. If you find yourself unsure about any dietary adjustments or if you encounter any symptoms, please consult with your healthcare provider. Your doctor or a registered dietitian can provide personalized guidance based on your medical history and current health status, ensuring that you make the best choices for your well-being.

Additionally, while we have provided nutritional information for each recipe to help you make informed decisions, please note that these values are approximate. Variations in ingredients, portion sizes, and cooking methods can all impact the final nutritional content of your meals. Therefore, use the nutritional information as a general guide rather than an exact measure.

Furthermore, If our cookbook has brought joy to your kitchen and table, we'd be thrilled to hear about your experiences in an Amazon review. On the flip side, if you stumble upon any hiccups while exploring our recipes, don't hesitate to get in touch at **kloppkingsley@gmail.com.** We're here to support your cooking journey every step of the way.

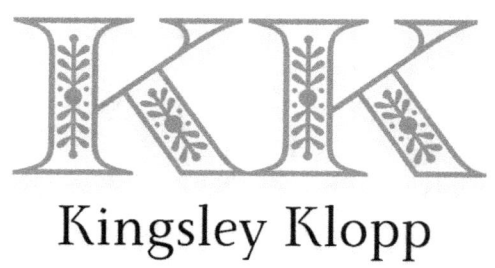

Introduction.

Welcome to the **Pancreatitis Diet Cookbook for Seniors**, an abundance of delectable and healthful meals designed specifically for those navigating the challenges of living with pancreatitis. If you've picked up this book, you likely know the struggle all too well—dealing with the pain, discomfort, and dietary restrictions that come with managing pancreatitis. But here's the good news: you can still enjoy flavorful, satisfying meals that support your health and well-being. This cookbook is your guide to discovering just how enjoyable and fulfilling a pancreatitis-friendly diet can be. Living with pancreatitis often means making significant changes to your diet, but these changes don't have to be daunting or dull. In fact, with the right recipes and a bit of creativity, you'll find that healthy eating can be both delicious and exciting.

This cookbook is packed with easy-to-follow recipes that cater to your nutritional needs while tantalizing your taste buds. From hearty breakfasts to energizing lunches and comforting dinners, you'll find a wide variety of meals that are not only good for your pancreas but also for your overall health. We understand that as a senior, you may have specific dietary requirements and preferences, and this book is tailored to meet those needs. Each recipe is carefully crafted to be gentle on your digestive system while providing the essential nutrients your body needs. We focus on using fresh, wholesome ingredients that are low in fat and easy to digest, ensuring that you can enjoy each meal without worrying about triggering your symptoms. But this book is more than just a collection of recipes; it's a comprehensive guide to living well with pancreatitis. We'll walk you through the basics of pancreatitis, explaining what it is, how it affects your body, and why diet is such a crucial part of managing the condition. You'll learn about the foods to avoid and the ones to embrace, as well as practical tips for meal planning, shopping, and cooking.

Our goal is to empower you with the knowledge and tools you need to take control of your diet and your health. We want to show you that eating well doesn't have to be a chore—it can be a joy. By making smart food choices and trying new recipes, you can improve your quality of life, reduce your symptoms, and feel more energetic and vibrant every day.

One of the highlights of this cookbook is the variety of recipes that cater to different tastes and dietary needs. Whether you're a fan of savory dishes, sweet treats, or something in between, you'll find plenty of options to suit your palate. From simple snacks to gourmet dinners, each recipe is designed to be easy to prepare, using ingredients that are readily available and affordable. We've also included nutritional information for each dish, so you can keep track of your intake and make informed choices about what you eat. As you embark on this culinary journey, remember that you're not alone. Many people are successfully managing pancreatitis through diet, and you can too. This cookbook is here to support you every step of the way, providing you with delicious recipes, helpful tips, and the encouragement you need to stay committed to your health goals.

So, let's get cooking! Dive into the **Pancreatitis Diet Cookbook for Seniors** and discover a world of flavors that are as good for your taste buds as they are for your pancreas. Here's to your health, happiness, and culinary adventure. Enjoy every bite!

Chapter 1: Navigating Dietary Needs for Seniors

Nutritional Needs for Seniors

As we age, our bodies undergo numerous changes that impact our nutritional needs. For seniors, eating a balanced and nutritious diet is not just about maintaining physical health; it's about enhancing the quality of life, preserving independence, and enjoying each day to its fullest.

The Importance of Proper Nutrition
Imagine waking up every day feeling energized and ready to embrace whatever comes your way. Good nutrition is the key to unlocking this vitality. As seniors, our bodies require fewer calories, but they need more of certain nutrients to maintain health, support cognitive function, and keep chronic diseases at bay. Eating well can boost immunity, improve mental sharpness, and keep energy levels stable.

Key Nutrients for Seniors

1. Protein:
Protein is crucial for maintaining muscle mass and strength, which is essential for mobility and overall health. Seniors should include lean proteins like chicken, fish, beans, and legumes in their diets. For those who struggle with appetite or chewing, protein shakes or soft protein sources like eggs can be a great addition.

2. Fiber:
Fiber is vital for digestive health. It helps prevent constipation, which is a common issue as we age. Incorporating whole grains, fruits, vegetables, and legumes into daily meals can ensure adequate fiber intake, promoting regular bowel movements and a healthy gut.

3. Calcium and Vitamin D:
Bone health becomes a significant concern with age. Calcium and vitamin D work together to keep bones strong and prevent osteoporosis. Dairy products, leafy greens, and fortified foods are excellent sources. Don't forget about sunshine – spending a bit of time outdoors can boost vitamin D levels naturally.

4. Omega-3 Fatty Acids:
Omega-3s support heart health and cognitive function. Fatty fish like salmon, flaxseeds, and walnuts are rich in these beneficial fats. Including these in your diet can help reduce inflammation and support brain health, keeping your mind sharp and your heart healthy.

5. B Vitamins:
B vitamins, particularly B12, are essential for energy production and cognitive health. As we age, the body's ability to absorb B12 decreases, making it crucial to get enough from foods like meat, eggs, and dairy, or consider supplements if necessary.

6. Hydration:
Staying hydrated can sometimes be overlooked, yet it's vital for overall health. Dehydration can lead to confusion, urinary tract infections, and other serious issues. Aim to drink plenty of water throughout the day. Herbal teas, soups, and water-rich fruits like cucumbers and watermelon can also contribute to hydration.

Overcoming Common Challenges

Eating well in our later years isn't always easy. Appetite can decrease, and taste buds change, making food less appealing. Health conditions or medications can also impact what and how much we eat. Here are some tips to overcome these challenges:

- **Smaller, Frequent Meals:** Instead of three large meals, try eating smaller, more frequent meals. This can make eating less daunting and help maintain energy levels throughout the day.
- **Flavorful Foods**: Use herbs and spices to enhance the flavor of your meals. This can make food more enjoyable without adding extra salt or sugar.
- **Easy-to-Prepare Meals:** Simple, nutritious recipes can reduce the effort needed to eat well. Batch cooking and freezing portions can also make healthy eating more convenient.
- Social Eating: Sharing meals with family and friends can make eating a more enjoyable and meaningful experience. It can also provide emotional support and companionship.

Food is not just fuel; it is a source of comfort, a way to connect with loved ones, and a means to celebrate life's joys. For seniors, maintaining a healthy diet can foster a sense of independence and control over one's health. It can also bring back cherished memories of favorite meals and create new moments of joy and satisfaction. Taking the time to focus on nutrition is an act of self-love and care. It's about respecting the body that has carried you through life's journey and ensuring it continues to serve you well in the years to come. Remember, eating well is not about perfection; it's about making mindful choices that nourish both body and soul.

Common Dietary Challenges

Navigating the landscape of healthy eating can become increasingly complex as we age. Seniors face a unique set of dietary challenges that can impact their ability to maintain a balanced and nutritious diet. Understanding these challenges is the first step toward overcoming them and ensuring that our golden years are marked by vitality and well-being.

Changes in Appetite and Taste
As we age, our senses of taste and smell often diminish. Foods that once delighted our palates may now seem bland or unappetizing. This change can lead to a decreased interest in eating, resulting in inadequate nutrition. Additionally, a reduced sense of taste can cause seniors to add more salt or sugar to their meals, which can be detrimental to their health.
Solutions:
- Flavor Enhancements: Use herbs, spices, and natural flavorings to make meals more appealing without relying on salt or sugar.
- Variety: Incorporate a variety of foods to keep meals interesting and satisfying.
- Presentation: Pay attention to the visual appeal of food. Colorful, well-presented dishes can stimulate appetite.

Dental Issues
Dental problems such as missing teeth, gum disease, or dentures can make chewing difficult and painful. This can lead to a preference for softer, often less nutritious foods, and may cause some seniors to avoid eating altogether.
Solutions:
- Soft Foods: Incorporate soft, nutrient-dense foods such as yogurt, scrambled eggs, cooked vegetables, and smoothies.
- Dental Care: Regular dental check-ups and proper oral hygiene can help manage and prevent dental issues.

Digestive Changes
Aging can slow down the digestive system, leading to issues such as constipation, bloating, and reduced nutrient absorption. Medications commonly used by seniors can also affect digestion and appetite.
Solutions:
- Fiber: Increase fiber intake with whole grains, fruits, vegetables, and legumes to promote digestive health.
- Hydration: Ensure adequate fluid intake to help with digestion and prevent constipation.
- Probiotics: Incorporate probiotic-rich foods like yogurt and kefir to support gut health.

Chronic Health Conditions

Chronic conditions such as diabetes, heart disease, and hypertension are more common in seniors and often require dietary restrictions. Managing these conditions through diet can be challenging, especially when multiple restrictions overlap.

Solutions:
- Tailored Diet Plans: Work with a healthcare provider or nutritionist to create a diet plan that accommodates all health conditions.
- Balanced Approach: Focus on nutrient-dense foods that can meet dietary restrictions while providing essential nutrients.

Medication Interactions

Medications can interfere with appetite, taste, and nutrient absorption. Some drugs can cause side effects such as dry mouth, nausea, or altered taste, which can deter seniors from eating well.

Solutions:
- Medical Guidance: Consult with healthcare providers about potential side effects and possible alternatives.
- Hydration and Snacks: Encourage small, frequent meals and adequate hydration to combat side effects.

Social and Emotional Factors

Eating is often a social activity, and seniors may face loneliness or isolation, leading to a lack of motivation to prepare and eat balanced meals. Depression and anxiety can also negatively impact appetite and dietary habits.

Solutions:
- Social Meals: Encourage shared meals with family and friends to make eating a more enjoyable and social experience.
- Community Programs: Participate in community meal programs or senior centers that offer nutritious meals and social interaction.
- Mental Health Support: Address underlying emotional issues with professional support and counseling if needed.

Financial Constraints

Many seniors live on fixed incomes and may struggle to afford healthy, fresh foods. This financial strain can lead to reliance on cheaper, processed foods that are often less nutritious.

Solutions:
- Budget-Friendly Options: Focus on affordable, nutrient-dense foods like beans, lentils, frozen vegetables, and whole grains.
- Assistance Programs: Utilize food assistance programs like SNAP (Supplemental Nutrition Assistance Program) or local food banks.

Mobility and Convenience

Limited mobility and physical limitations can make grocery shopping and meal preparation difficult. Seniors may find it challenging to stand for long periods or to handle heavy pots and pans.

Solutions:
- Convenient Options: Use pre-chopped vegetables, pre-cooked grains, and other convenience foods that are still healthy.
- Meal Services: Consider meal delivery services that provide balanced, ready-to-eat meals tailored to seniors' dietary needs.
- Adaptive Equipment: Use kitchen tools designed to aid those with limited strength or dexterity.

Tips for Maintaining a Healthy Diet

1. Prioritize Nutrient-Dense Foods

As calorie needs decrease with age, it's essential to focus on nutrient-dense foods that provide vitamins, minerals, and other essential nutrients without excess calories.

- Fruits and Vegetables: Aim for a colorful variety of fruits and vegetables, which are rich in vitamins, minerals, and antioxidants. Fresh, frozen, or canned options (without added sugar or salt) are all good choices.
- Whole Grains: Choose whole grains like brown rice, quinoa, oats, and whole wheat bread over refined grains. Whole grains are higher in fiber, which is important for digestive health.
- Lean Proteins: Include sources of lean protein such as chicken, turkey, fish, beans, lentils, and tofu. Protein is crucial for maintaining muscle mass and strength.
- Healthy Fats: Incorporate healthy fats from sources like avocados, nuts, seeds, and olive oil. These fats support brain health and can help manage cholesterol levels.

2. Stay Hydrated

Dehydration is a common issue among seniors, as the sense of thirst diminishes with age. Adequate hydration is vital for overall health, aiding in digestion, nutrient absorption, and joint lubrication.

- Water: Aim to drink at least 8 glasses of water a day. Carry a water bottle and take small sips throughout the day.
- Hydrating Foods: Include water-rich foods like cucumbers, watermelon, oranges, and soups.
- Limit Diuretics: Reduce the intake of caffeine and alcohol, which can contribute to dehydration.

3. Eat Regular, Balanced Meals

Skipping meals can lead to energy dips and nutrient deficiencies. Eating regular, balanced meals helps maintain steady energy levels and ensures a consistent intake of essential nutrients.

- Small, Frequent Meals: If large meals are overwhelming, try eating smaller, more frequent meals and snacks throughout the day.
- Balanced Plates: Aim to fill half your plate with fruits and vegetables, a quarter with lean protein, and a quarter with whole grains.

4. Incorporate Fiber-Rich Foods

Fiber is crucial for digestive health and can help prevent constipation, which is a common issue in seniors.

- Whole Grains: Choose whole grain bread, cereals, and pasta.
- Fruits and Vegetables: Include high-fiber fruits like apples, pears, and berries, and vegetables like carrots, broccoli, and leafy greens.
- Legumes: Beans, lentils, and chickpeas are excellent sources of fiber.

5. Monitor and Manage Portion Sizes

Eating appropriate portion sizes can help manage weight and prevent overeating, which is particularly important as metabolism slows with age.

- **Use Smaller Plates:** Smaller plates can help control portion sizes and prevent overeating.
- **Mindful Eating:** Pay attention to hunger and fullness cues, and eat slowly to give your body time to signal when it's satisfied.

6. Enhance Flavor Without Extra Salt or Sugar

As taste buds change with age, it's common to add more salt or sugar to enhance flavor. However, excessive salt and sugar can lead to health issues like hypertension and diabetes.

- **Herbs and Spices:** Use herbs, spices, and citrus to add flavor without extra salt or sugar. Experiment with basil, rosemary, turmeric, and lemon zest.
- **Naturally Sweet Foods:** Opt for naturally sweet foods like fruits to satisfy sweet cravings.

7. Plan and Prepare Meals Ahead

Planning and preparing meals ahead of time can make healthy eating more manageable and reduce reliance on convenience foods, which are often less nutritious.

- **Weekly Meal Plans:** Create a weekly meal plan that includes a variety of nutrient-dense foods. This can simplify grocery shopping and ensure balanced meals.
- **Batch Cooking:** Cook larger portions of meals and freeze leftovers for days when cooking feels like a chore.
- **Easy Recipes:** Focus on simple, easy-to-prepare recipes that don't require extensive time or effort.

8. Make Mealtime Enjoyable

Mealtime should be a pleasant experience, not a chore. Creating an enjoyable mealtime environment can enhance appetite and improve overall nutrition.

- **Social Meals:** Share meals with family and friends when possible. Eating with others can make meals more enjoyable and provide social interaction.
- **Ambiance:** Set the table nicely, play soft music, and create a calm and pleasant dining environment.

9. Address Special Dietary Needs

Seniors often have specific dietary needs or restrictions due to health conditions. It's essential to tailor the diet to these needs while still ensuring it is balanced and nutritious.

- **Consult Professionals:** Work with a nutritionist or healthcare provider to create a diet plan that meets individual health needs.
- **Read Labels:** Pay attention to food labels to avoid ingredients that may exacerbate health conditions.

10. Stay Physically Active

Physical activity complements a healthy diet by promoting overall health, maintaining muscle mass, and supporting metabolism.

- Regular Exercise: Engage in regular physical activities like walking, swimming, or yoga. Even light exercise can make a significant difference.
- Combine with Social Activities: Join exercise classes or groups to combine physical activity with social interaction.

Chapter 2: Understanding Pancreatitis

Types of Pancreatitis: Acute vs. Chronic

Acute Pancreatitis: An Unexpected Storm
What It Is: Acute pancreatitis is a sudden inflammation of the pancreas, a small but vital gland located behind the stomach. The pancreas plays a crucial role in digestion and blood sugar regulation, producing enzymes and hormones essential for breaking down food and managing glucose levels. When the pancreas becomes inflamed, its enzymes start digesting the gland itself, leading to severe pain and swelling.

Symptoms: The onset of acute pancreatitis is often abrupt and intense, manifesting through:
- Severe Abdominal Pain: This pain typically starts in the upper abdomen and can radiate to the back. It's often described as a burning or stabbing sensation, making it difficult to sit still or find comfort.
- Nausea and Vomiting: The inflammation can trigger relentless nausea and vomiting, exacerbating the discomfort and dehydration.
- Fever: The body's response to inflammation may include a fever, signaling the immune system's fight against the problem.
- Rapid Pulse: An elevated heart rate is common due to pain and inflammation.

Causes: Common causes include gallstones, which block the pancreatic duct, and excessive alcohol consumption. Other triggers can be certain medications, infections, or trauma to the abdomen.

Emotional Impact: Experiencing acute pancreatitis can be frightening and disorienting. The sudden, intense pain and urgent medical intervention required can leave individuals feeling vulnerable and anxious about their health. The need for immediate hospitalization adds to the emotional strain, as patients grapple with fear, uncertainty, and the abrupt disruption of their lives.

Treatment:
- Hospitalization: Most cases require hospitalization to manage pain, administer intravenous fluids, and monitor complications.
- Fasting: Patients are often advised to fast initially to allow the pancreas to rest.
- Medications: Pain relief and antibiotics may be administered as needed.
- Long-Term Care: Addressing underlying causes, such as gallstone removal or lifestyle changes to reduce alcohol consumption, is essential.

Chronic Pancreatitis: A Lingering Battle

What It Is: Chronic pancreatitis is a long-term inflammation of the pancreas that gradually damages its structure and function. Unlike the sudden onset of acute pancreatitis, chronic pancreatitis develops over time, leading to permanent damage and scarring of the pancreas.

Symptoms: Chronic pancreatitis often presents a different set of challenges, including:
- Persistent Abdominal Pain: This pain is usually less intense than acute pancreatitis but can be constant and debilitating, significantly affecting daily life.
- Digestive Issues: The damaged pancreas struggles to produce digestive enzymes, leading to malabsorption, diarrhea, and weight loss.
- Diabetes: The pancreas's impaired ability to produce insulin can result in diabetes, adding another layer of complexity to management.

Causes: Long-term alcohol abuse is the most common cause, but chronic pancreatitis can also result from genetic factors, autoimmune diseases, or recurrent episodes of acute pancreatitis. Certain conditions, like cystic fibrosis, can also predispose individuals to chronic pancreatitis.

Emotional Impact: Living with chronic pancreatitis requires enduring persistent pain and managing ongoing health issues, which can be emotionally exhausting. The chronic nature of the condition often leads to feelings of frustration, helplessness, and anxiety about the future. It demands constant vigilance over diet and lifestyle, potentially leading to social isolation and a diminished quality of life.

Treatment:
- Pain Management: Long-term pain relief strategies, including medications and nerve blocks, are often necessary.
- Enzyme Supplements: Pancreatic enzyme supplements can aid digestion and improve nutrient absorption.
- Lifestyle Changes: Abstaining from alcohol, adopting a low-fat diet, and quitting smoking are crucial steps.
- Medical Interventions: In some cases, surgery or endoscopic procedures may be needed to alleviate obstructions or manage complications.

Both acute and chronic pancreatitis demand resilience and adaptability. The physical pain is accompanied by emotional challenges that can test one's spirit and willpower. However, with the right medical care, lifestyle adjustments, and support system, managing pancreatitis becomes possible.

Support Systems:
- Healthcare Team: Regular consultations with gastroenterologists, nutritionists, and pain specialists are essential.
- Support Groups: Connecting with others who understand the journey can provide emotional support and practical advice.
- Family and Friends: Leaning on loved ones for support can make a significant difference in coping with the day-to-day challenges.

Symptoms and Diagnosis of Pancreatitis

Symptoms of Pancreatitis

Pancreatitis manifests differently depending on whether it is acute or chronic. Recognizing these symptoms is the first step towards seeking appropriate medical care.

Acute Pancreatitis: Acute pancreatitis is characterized by a sudden onset of symptoms that can range from mild to severe. Common symptoms include:
- Severe Abdominal Pain: The hallmark symptom of acute pancreatitis is intense pain in the upper abdomen, often radiating to the back. This pain can appear suddenly and persist for several days, becoming worse after eating or drinking, especially fatty foods.
- Nausea and Vomiting: Alongside the pain, acute pancreatitis frequently causes nausea and vomiting, which can exacerbate dehydration and weakness.
- Fever: The body's inflammatory response can lead to a high fever, indicating the severity of the condition.
- Rapid Pulse: An elevated heart rate is often observed due to pain and the body's stress response.
- Tenderness When Touching the Abdomen: The abdominal area may be extremely sensitive to touch, adding to the discomfort.

Chronic Pancreatitis: Chronic pancreatitis develops over time, with symptoms that may be less severe but more persistent and debilitating. Common symptoms include:
- Chronic Abdominal Pain: Pain in chronic pancreatitis can be constant or episodic, often felt in the upper abdomen and radiating to the back. It may worsen after meals and become increasingly difficult to manage over time.
- Digestive Problems: The pancreas's impaired ability to produce digestive enzymes leads to symptoms like bloating, gas, diarrhea, and oily stools (steatorrhea), indicating malabsorption of fats and nutrients.
- Weight Loss: Unintended weight loss occurs due to the body's inability to absorb nutrients properly, compounded by a reduced appetite and ongoing digestive issues.
- Jaundice: Yellowing of the skin and eyes can occur if bile ducts become blocked by inflammation or scarring.
- Diabetes: Chronic inflammation of the pancreas can damage insulin-producing cells, leading to diabetes.

Diagnosis of Pancreatitis

Diagnosing pancreatitis involves a combination of clinical evaluation, laboratory tests, and imaging studies. Accurate diagnosis is essential for determining the appropriate treatment and managing the condition effectively.

Clinical Evaluation: The first step in diagnosing pancreatitis is a thorough medical history and physical examination by a healthcare provider. Key points include:
- Symptom Description: Detailed accounts of the nature, onset, and duration of abdominal pain, digestive issues, and other related symptoms.
- Medical History: History of alcohol use, gallstones, previous episodes of pancreatitis, and family history of pancreatic diseases.
- Physical Examination: Assessment of abdominal tenderness, distension, and other signs of systemic illness.

Laboratory Tests: Blood tests are crucial for diagnosing pancreatitis and evaluating its severity. Common tests include:
- Amylase and Lipase Levels: Elevated levels of these pancreatic enzymes in the blood are strong indicators of acute pancreatitis.
- Liver Function Tests: Abnormal results can suggest bile duct obstruction or concurrent liver disease.
- Blood Glucose Levels: High glucose levels can indicate damage to insulin-producing cells in the pancreas, common in chronic pancreatitis.
- Complete Blood Count (CBC): Can reveal signs of infection, inflammation, or other related conditions.
- Electrolyte Levels: To check for imbalances that may result from vomiting and dehydration.

Imaging Studies: Imaging is essential for visualizing the pancreas and detecting complications. Common imaging tests include:
- Ultrasound: Often the first imaging test performed, particularly useful for detecting gallstones.
- CT Scan (Computed Tomography): Provides detailed images of the pancreas and surrounding organs, helping to identify inflammation, necrosis, or fluid collections.
- MRI (Magnetic Resonance Imaging): Offers detailed images of the pancreas, ducts, and surrounding tissues, useful for diagnosing chronic pancreatitis.
- Endoscopic Ultrasound (EUS): Combines endoscopy and ultrasound to provide detailed images and is particularly useful for detecting small abnormalities.
- ERCP (Endoscopic Retrograde Cholangiopancreatography): An advanced endoscopic procedure to visualize the bile and pancreatic ducts, often used if a blockage is suspected.

Emotional and Practical Considerations

Facing the symptoms and undergoing the diagnostic process for pancreatitis can be an emotionally challenging experience. The sudden, severe pain of acute pancreatitis or the persistent discomfort and digestive issues of chronic pancreatitis can lead to anxiety, stress, and feelings of helplessness.

Emotional Support:

- Seek Support: Reach out to family, friends, or support groups to share your experiences and feelings. Knowing that others understand and care can provide significant comfort.
- Professional Counseling: Consider speaking with a mental health professional to manage stress, anxiety, or depression that may accompany chronic illness.

Practical Steps:

- Follow Medical Advice: Adhere to treatment plans and dietary recommendations provided by healthcare professionals to manage symptoms and prevent complications.
- Stay Informed: Educate yourself about pancreatitis to understand your condition better and make informed decisions about your health care.
- Healthy Lifestyle Choices: Adopt lifestyle changes such as reducing alcohol intake, quitting smoking, and maintaining a balanced diet to support pancreatic health.

Impact of Pancreatitis on Digestion

The Role of the Pancreas in Digestion
The pancreas is a vital gland situated behind the stomach, playing a dual role in the digestive and endocrine systems. Its primary functions include:
- **Enzyme Production**: The pancreas produces digestive enzymes, such as amylase, lipase, and proteases, which are essential for breaking down carbohydrates, fats, and proteins in the small intestine.
- **Hormone Secretion**: It secretes insulin and glucagon, hormones that regulate blood sugar levels.

When pancreatitis strikes, these critical functions are compromised, leading to a range of digestive problems.

Acute Pancreatitis and Digestion
Immediate Disruption: In acute pancreatitis, the inflammation is sudden and severe. The digestive enzymes that the pancreas normally secretes into the small intestine start attacking the pancreas itself. This auto-digestion leads to:
- **Severe Abdominal Pain**: The intense pain can make eating and digestion almost unbearable.
- **Nausea and Vomiting**: These symptoms are common and can prevent food intake, leading to dehydration and nutritional deficiencies.

Short-term Effects: During an acute episode, the digestive process is significantly impaired:
- **Reduced Enzyme Production**: The inflamed pancreas cannot produce enough enzymes, leading to poor digestion and nutrient absorption.
- **Bile Duct Obstruction**: Inflammation can block the bile duct, preventing bile from aiding in fat digestion.

Emotional Toll: The sudden onset and severity of symptoms can be frightening and overwhelming. The pain, combined with the inability to eat normally, can lead to feelings of frustration and helplessness.

Chronic Pancreatitis and Digestion
Persistent Challenges: Chronic pancreatitis develops gradually, leading to ongoing inflammation and progressive damage to the pancreas. This chronic condition has a more prolonged and profound impact on digestion:
- **Continuous Abdominal Pain**: Persistent or recurrent pain can significantly affect appetite and willingness to eat.
- **Malabsorption**: The chronic inflammation leads to a continuous reduction in digestive enzyme production, resulting in poor digestion and nutrient absorption.
- **Steatorrhea**: Fat malabsorption causes oily, foul-smelling stools that float (steatorrhea). This is a clear sign that fats are not being properly digested and absorbed.

Long-term Effects: Over time, the cumulative damage to the pancreas exacerbates digestive issues:
- **Nutritional Deficiencies:** Poor absorption of nutrients leads to deficiencies in vitamins and minerals, causing weight loss, muscle wasting, and overall weakness.
- **Diabetes:** Chronic pancreatitis can damage the insulin-producing cells, leading to diabetes, which further complicates dietary management.

Emotional Impact: Living with chronic pancreatitis is emotionally draining. The persistent pain, constant dietary restrictions, and fear of flare-ups can lead to anxiety, depression, and social isolation. The need to constantly monitor food intake and the frequent digestive discomfort can overshadow daily life.

Managing Digestive Issues

Dietary Adjustments: Proper diet management is key to alleviating digestive issues related to pancreatitis:
- Low-fat Diet: Since fat digestion is impaired, a low-fat diet can reduce symptoms and improve nutrient absorption. Opt for lean proteins, whole grains, and plenty of fruits and vegetables.
- Small, Frequent Meals: Eating smaller meals more frequently can ease the digestive burden on the pancreas.
- Enzyme Supplements: Pancreatic enzyme replacement therapy (PERT) can aid digestion and nutrient absorption, improving symptoms like steatorrhea and malnutrition.
- Hydration: Adequate fluid intake is crucial to support overall health and digestion.

Medical Management:
- Pain Relief: Managing pain through medications or other therapies is essential for improving quality of life.
- Nutritional Support: Working with a dietitian or nutritionist can help tailor a diet plan that meets individual nutritional needs and preferences.

Emotional Support:
- Counseling: Psychological support can help manage the emotional toll of chronic illness. Therapy or counseling can provide coping strategies and emotional resilience.
- Support Groups: Connecting with others who understand the challenges of pancreatitis can provide comfort, practical advice, and a sense of community.

Foods to Avoid

Managing pancreatitis requires careful attention to diet. Certain foods can exacerbate symptoms and lead to flare-ups, while others can help support pancreatic health and overall well-being. Knowing which foods to avoid is crucial for managing both acute and chronic pancreatitis, as it can help prevent pain, inflammation, and other digestive issues.

High-Fat Foods
The pancreas plays a key role in breaking down fats. When it is inflamed or damaged, its ability to produce enzymes for fat digestion is compromised. Consuming high-fat foods can place additional strain on the pancreas, leading to increased pain and discomfort.
Foods to Avoid:
- Fried Foods: French fries, fried chicken, doughnuts, and other deep-fried items are high in unhealthy fats and can trigger pancreatitis symptoms.
- Fatty Cuts of Meat: Sausages, bacon, ribs, and fatty cuts of beef, pork, and lamb contain high levels of saturated fats.
- Full-Fat Dairy Products: Whole milk, cream, butter, cheese, and full-fat yogurt are rich in saturated fats.
- Pastries and Desserts: Cakes, cookies, pastries, and ice cream often contain high levels of both fats and sugars.

Impact on Digestion: High-fat foods are difficult to digest without adequate enzyme production, leading to symptoms like abdominal pain, bloating, and steatorrhea (oily, foul-smelling stools). They can also trigger acute pancreatitis episodes and worsen chronic pancreatitis.

Sugary Foods and Beverages
High sugar intake can lead to increased insulin demand, stressing an already compromised pancreas, especially in chronic pancreatitis, where the risk of diabetes is higher.
Foods to Avoid:
- Sugary Drinks: Sodas, energy drinks, sweetened coffee and tea, and fruit juices with added sugar are high in sugar and can contribute to inflammation.
- Sweets and Candies: Candy bars, gummies, chocolates, and other sweets are loaded with sugar.
- Processed Snacks: Many packaged snacks, including granola bars, flavored yogurts, and breakfast cereals, contain high levels of added sugars.

Impact on Digestion: Excessive sugar can lead to spikes in blood sugar levels, increasing the risk of diabetes. High sugar intake can also contribute to weight gain, further complicating pancreatitis management.

Alcohol

Alcohol is a significant risk factor for both acute and chronic pancreatitis. It can cause inflammation of the pancreas and increase the risk of recurrent episodes.

Foods to Avoid:
- Alcoholic Beverages: Beer, wine, spirits, and cocktails should be completely avoided.

Impact on Digestion: Alcohol irritates the pancreas and can cause enzyme activation within the pancreas itself, leading to self-digestion and severe inflammation. Chronic alcohol consumption can lead to permanent pancreatic damage.

Processed and Red Meats

Processed and red meats are high in saturated fats and often contain additives and preservatives that can be harmful to the pancreas.

Foods to Avoid:
- Processed Meats: Sausages, hot dogs, deli meats, and bacon contain unhealthy fats and additives.
- Red Meats: Beef, lamb, and pork, especially fatty cuts, should be limited or avoided.

Impact on Digestion: These meats can trigger inflammation and are difficult for the pancreas to break down, leading to digestive discomfort and exacerbating pancreatitis symptoms.

High-Sodium Foods

High-sodium diets can increase blood pressure and put additional strain on the pancreas and other organs.

Foods to Avoid:
- Processed and Packaged Foods: Canned soups, instant noodles, frozen meals, and other processed foods are often high in sodium.
- Salty Snacks: Chips, pretzels, and salted nuts contain high levels of sodium.

Impact on Digestion: High sodium intake can lead to fluid retention and increased blood pressure, which can complicate pancreatitis management and overall health.

Spicy Foods

Spicy foods can irritate the digestive tract and exacerbate symptoms of pancreatitis, including pain and inflammation.

Foods to Avoid:
- Hot Peppers and Spices: Chili peppers, hot sauce, and dishes heavily spiced with cayenne or other hot spices should be limited.
- Spicy Condiments: Mustard, horseradish, and other spicy condiments can also cause irritation.

Impact on Digestion: Spicy foods can increase stomach acid production and irritate the gastrointestinal lining, leading to increased pain and discomfort.

High-Fiber Raw Vegetables and Fruits

While fiber is generally good for digestion, certain high-fiber foods can be difficult for those with pancreatitis to digest, especially in raw form.

Foods to Avoid:
- Raw Vegetables: Broccoli, cauliflower, cabbage, and Brussels sprouts can cause bloating and gas.
- Raw Fruits: Apples, pears, and berries with seeds can be difficult to digest and may lead to discomfort.

Impact on Digestion: High-fiber foods, when not cooked, can lead to bloating, gas, and discomfort, exacerbating pancreatitis symptoms.

Hence, avoiding certain foods is crucial for managing pancreatitis and maintaining a healthy digestive system. By steering clear of high-fat, sugary, and processed foods, alcohol, high-sodium items, spicy dishes, and certain high-fiber raw vegetables and fruits, individuals with pancreatitis can reduce inflammation and digestive discomfort.

Foods to Include

Lean Proteins
Proteins are essential for healing and maintaining muscle mass, but it's crucial to choose lean sources that are easier on the pancreas.
Foods to Include:
- Poultry: Skinless chicken and turkey are excellent sources of lean protein.
- Fish: Fatty fish like salmon, mackerel, and sardines are rich in omega-3 fatty acids, which have anti-inflammatory properties. However, they should be consumed in moderation to avoid high-fat intake.
- Eggs: Egg whites are a good source of protein without the fat found in yolks.
- Legumes: Beans, lentils, and chickpeas provide plant-based protein and fiber.
- Low-Fat Dairy: Skim milk, low-fat yogurt, and low-fat cheese provide protein and calcium without excessive fat.

Benefits: Lean proteins help repair tissues and support immune function without adding unnecessary fat that can strain the pancreas.

Whole Grains
Whole grains are rich in fiber, vitamins, and minerals, and they support digestive health and stable blood sugar levels.
Foods to Include:
- Oats: A great source of soluble fiber that can help with digestion.
- Brown Rice: A whole grain that provides fiber and essential nutrients.
- Quinoa: A protein-rich grain that is also high in fiber.
- Whole Wheat Bread and Pasta: Better options than refined grains as they contain more nutrients and fiber.

Benefits: Whole grains aid digestion, promote satiety, and provide sustained energy levels, making them ideal for managing pancreatitis.

Fruits and Vegetables
Fruits and vegetables are packed with essential vitamins, minerals, and antioxidants that support overall health and reduce inflammation.
Foods to Include:
- Cooked Vegetables: Steamed or roasted vegetables like carrots, zucchini, spinach, and sweet potatoes are easier to digest and less likely to cause bloating.
- Non-Acidic Fruits: Applesauce, bananas, berries, and melons are gentle on the digestive system.
- Leafy Greens: Spinach, kale, and Swiss chard are nutrient-dense and can be cooked to improve digestibility.

Benefits: Fruits and vegetables provide vital nutrients and antioxidants that help reduce inflammation and support overall health. Cooking vegetables makes them easier to digest, which is beneficial for those with pancreatitis.

Healthy Fats

While fat intake should be limited, incorporating small amounts of healthy fats is essential for overall health.

Foods to Include:
- Avocados: A good source of healthy monounsaturated fats and fiber.
- Nuts and Seeds: Almonds, walnuts, chia seeds, and flaxseeds provide omega-3 fatty acids and protein. Consume in moderation and choose unsalted varieties.
- Olive Oil: A heart-healthy fat that can be used in cooking or as a salad dressing.

Benefits: Healthy fats support heart health and reduce inflammation without overburdening the pancreas. Consuming these fats in moderation ensures they contribute positively to your diet.

Low-Fat Dairy Products

Dairy is an important source of calcium and protein, but it's crucial to choose low-fat options to avoid putting stress on the pancreas.

Foods to Include:
- Skim Milk: Provides calcium and protein without the fat found in whole milk.
- Low-Fat Yogurt: Opt for plain, low-fat yogurt that is lower in fat and added sugars.
- Low-Fat Cheese: Choose options like low-fat cottage cheese or part-skim mozzarella.

Benefits: Low-fat dairy products offer the benefits of dairy without the high fat content that can exacerbate pancreatitis symptoms.

Hydrating Foods and Beverages

Staying hydrated is crucial for overall health and digestive function.

Foods to Include:
- Water: The best choice for hydration. Aim for at least 8 glasses a day.
- Herbal Teas: Chamomile, peppermint, and ginger teas can soothe the digestive system.
- Broth-Based Soups: Provide fluids and nutrients without added fat.
- Water-Rich Fruits and Vegetables: Cucumbers, watermelon, and oranges help with hydration.

Benefits: Proper hydration supports digestion, helps prevent constipation, and keeps the body functioning optimally.

Anti-Inflammatory Foods

Incorporating foods with natural anti-inflammatory properties can help reduce pancreatic inflammation.

Foods to Include:
- Turmeric: Contains curcumin, which has strong anti-inflammatory effects.
- Ginger: Known for its digestive benefits and anti-inflammatory properties.
- Garlic: Can help reduce inflammation and boost the immune system.
- Berries: Blueberries, strawberries, and raspberries are rich in antioxidants and anti-inflammatory compounds.

Benefits: Anti-inflammatory foods help manage and reduce inflammation in the pancreas, aiding in the overall management of pancreatitis.

Practical Tips for Including These Foods

1. Meal Planning: Plan your meals to ensure they include a balance of lean proteins, whole grains, fruits, vegetables, and healthy fats. This can help manage portion sizes and ensure a variety of nutrients.
2. Cooking Methods: Opt for baking, steaming, grilling, or roasting instead of frying. These methods reduce fat content and preserve nutrients.
3. Snack Wisely: Choose healthy snacks like fresh fruit, yogurt, or a handful of nuts to maintain energy levels and avoid overeating during meals.
4. Read Labels: Check food labels for added sugars and unhealthy fats. Aim for natural, minimally processed foods.
5. Stay Hydrated: Drink plenty of water throughout the day and include water-rich foods to help with hydration.

Reading Food Labels

Why Reading Food Labels is Important
For individuals with pancreatitis, monitoring fat, sugar, and sodium intake is crucial to avoid triggering symptoms and to ensure overall health. Food labels help you:
- Identify hidden sources of fats, sugars, and sodium.
- Compare products to choose the healthiest options.
- Understand serving sizes and nutritional content.

Key Components of a Food Label

1. Serving Size and Servings Per Container: The serving size indicates the amount of food that is considered one serving. All nutritional information on the label is based on this serving size.
   - Importance: Pay attention to serving sizes to understand how much you are actually consuming. If you eat more than the serving size, you need to adjust the nutritional values accordingly.

2. Calories: Calories provide a measure of how much energy you get from a serving of food.
   - Importance: Monitoring calorie intake can help manage weight, which is important for overall health and managing pancreatitis symptoms.

3. Total Fat, Saturated Fat, and Trans Fat:
   - Total Fat: Indicates the total amount of fat in one serving.
   - Saturated Fat: A type of fat that should be limited as it can raise cholesterol levels and exacerbate pancreatitis symptoms.
   - Trans Fat: Unhealthy fats that should be avoided completely.
   - Importance: For pancreatitis, it is essential to limit total fat, particularly saturated and trans fats. Look for foods with low levels of these fats.

4. Cholesterol: The amount of cholesterol in a serving.
   - Importance: High cholesterol can contribute to gallstone formation, which can trigger pancreatitis. Choose foods with lower cholesterol levels.

5. Sodium: Indicates the amount of salt in a serving.
   - Importance: High sodium intake can lead to increased blood pressure and fluid retention, complicating pancreatitis management. Aim for low-sodium options.

6. Total Carbohydrates, Dietary Fiber, and Sugars:
   - Total Carbohydrates: Includes all types of carbohydrates, including sugars and dietary fiber.
   - Dietary Fiber: Essential for digestive health. Higher fiber is generally better.
   - Sugars: Includes natural and added sugars.
   - Importance: Choose foods high in dietary fiber and low in added sugars to support digestion and maintain stable blood sugar levels.
7. Protein: The amount of protein in one serving.
   - Importance: Protein is essential for healing and maintaining muscle mass, but it should come from lean sources for those with pancreatitis.
8. Vitamins and Minerals: Information on important vitamins and minerals like Vitamin D, calcium, iron, and potassium.
   - Importance: Ensure you get enough essential nutrients to support overall health. Choose foods that provide beneficial vitamins and minerals.

The Ingredient List
The ingredient list provides a detailed account of everything included in the food product, listed in descending order by weight.
   - Importance: Understanding the ingredients helps you avoid those that might trigger pancreatitis symptoms or those that are unhealthy, such as high-fat ingredients, added sugars, and artificial additives.

Tips for Reading Food Labels
1. Look for Low-Fat Options:
   - What to Look For: Foods labeled as "low-fat," "reduced-fat," or "fat-free." However, ensure these do not compensate for fat with added sugars.
2. Avoid Added Sugars:
   - What to Look For: Ingredients like sucrose, high fructose corn syrup, molasses, and cane sugar. Choose foods with minimal added sugars.
3. Check for Low Sodium:
   - What to Look For: Foods labeled as "low-sodium," "reduced sodium," or "no added salt." Aim for products with less than 140 mg of sodium per serving.
4. Focus on Fiber:
   - What to Look For: Whole grains and foods high in dietary fiber, which aid digestion and help manage pancreatitis symptoms.
5. Beware of Trans Fats:
   - What to Look For: Partially hydrogenated oils in the ingredient list. Even if the label says "0g trans fat," it can still contain trans fats if partially hydrogenated oils are listed.
6. Pay Attention to Serving Sizes:
   - What to Look For: The serving size listed at the top of the label and compare it to your usual portion sizes to accurately gauge calorie and nutrient intake.

7. Compare Products:
   - What to Look For: Use the % Daily Value (%DV) to compare the nutrient content of similar products and choose the healthier option. Aim for lower %DV of fats, cholesterol, and sodium, and higher %DV of fiber, vitamins, and minerals.

Practical Examples

Example 1: Choosing Yogurt
   - Compare Brands: Look for yogurts that are low-fat or fat-free.
   - Check Sugars: Choose those with low or no added sugars. Greek yogurt is often a good choice for higher protein content with fewer added sugars.
   - Examine Ingredients: Avoid those with artificial flavors and sweeteners.

Example 2: Selecting Cereal
   - Fiber Content: Choose cereals with at least 3 grams of fiber per serving.
   - Sugar Content: Opt for cereals with less than 5 grams of sugar per serving.
   - Whole Grains: Ensure the first ingredient listed is a whole grain, such as whole oats or whole wheat.

In summary, reading food labels is a powerful tool in managing pancreatitis and maintaining overall health. By understanding and utilizing the information provided on labels, you can make informed decisions that support your dietary needs and help prevent flare-ups. Focus on low-fat, low-sugar, and low-sodium options, and prioritize foods high in dietary fiber and essential nutrients. This mindful approach to food selection will not only aid in managing pancreatitis but also promote long-term health and well-being.

Remember, every time you read a food label and choose a healthier option, you're taking a proactive step towards better managing your condition and improving your quality of life. With practice, reading labels becomes second nature, empowering you to make the best dietary choices with confidence.

Breakfast Recipes

1. Banana Oatmeal Porridge
Ingredients:
- 1 cup rolled oats
- 2 cups water or skim milk
- 1 ripe banana, mashed
- 1 tsp ground cinnamon
- 1 tsp vanilla extract
- 1 tbsp chia seeds
- 1 tbsp honey (optional)
- Fresh berries for topping (optional)

Instructions:
1. In a medium saucepan, bring the water or skim milk to a boil.
2. Add the rolled oats and reduce the heat to a simmer. Cook for about 5 minutes, stirring occasionally.
3. Stir in the mashed banana, ground cinnamon, vanilla extract, and chia seeds. Continue to cook for another 2-3 minutes until the oats are creamy and the banana is well incorporated.
4. Remove from heat and let sit for a minute.
5. Serve warm, topped with fresh berries and a drizzle of honey if desired.

Nutrition Info per Serving:
- Calories: 220
- Protein: 6g
- Carbohydrates: 45g
- Dietary Fiber: 7g
- Sugars: 12g
- Fat: 3g
- Saturated Fat: 0.5g
- Sodium: 10mg

Servings: 2
Cooking Time: 10 minutes

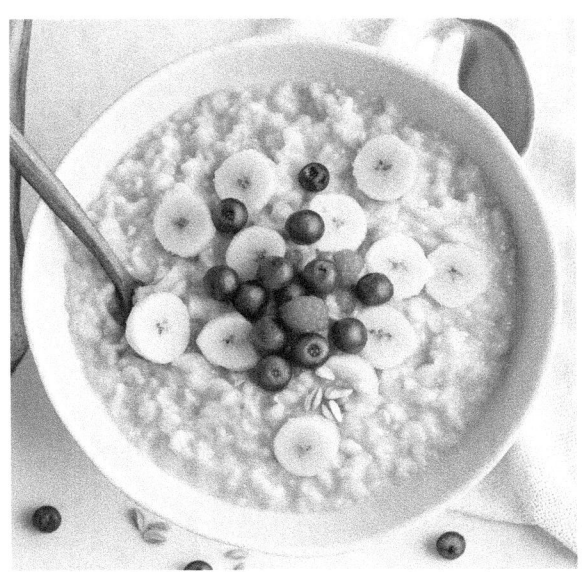

2. Smoothie Bowl

Ingredients:
- 1 cup unsweetened almond milk
- 1 cup frozen mixed berries
- 1 small banana
- 1 tbsp chia seeds
- 1 tbsp flaxseeds
- 1/2 cup Greek yogurt (fat-free)
- 1 tbsp honey (optional)
- Fresh fruit (e.g., sliced strawberries, blueberries) for topping
- 1 tbsp granola for topping

Instructions:
1. In a blender, combine the almond milk, frozen berries, banana, chia seeds, flaxseeds, Greek yogurt, and honey. Blend until smooth.
2. Pour the smoothie into a bowl.
3. Top with fresh fruit and granola.
4. Serve immediately.

Nutrition Info per Serving:
- Calories: 290
- Protein: 12g
- Carbohydrates: 48g
- Dietary Fiber: 10g
- Sugars: 25g
- Fat: 7g
- Saturated Fat: 0.5g
- Sodium: 60mg

Servings: 1
Cooking Time: 5 minutes

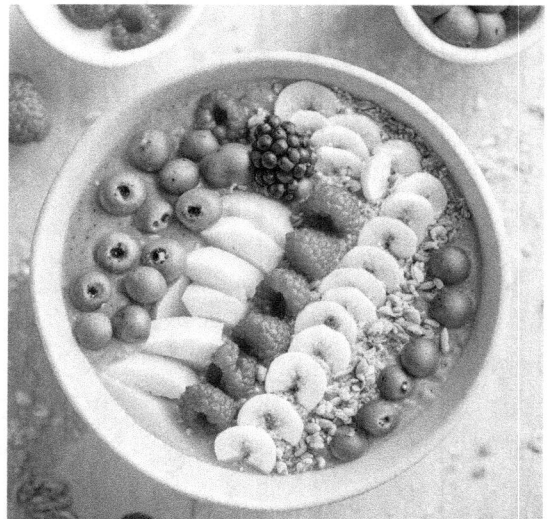

3. Egg White Scramble

Ingredients:
- 6 egg whites
- 1/4 cup skim milk
- 1 cup spinach, chopped
- 1/2 cup cherry tomatoes, halved
- 1/4 cup onion, finely chopped
- 1 tbsp olive oil
- 1/2 tsp ground black pepper
- 1/2 tsp garlic powder

Instructions:
1. In a medium bowl, whisk together the egg whites, skim milk, black pepper, and garlic powder.
2. Heat the olive oil in a non-stick skillet over medium heat.
3. Add the chopped onion and sauté for 2-3 minutes until translucent.
4. Add the spinach and cherry tomatoes, and cook for another 2 minutes until the spinach is wilted.
5. Pour the egg white mixture into the skillet, stirring gently until the eggs are fully cooked and scrambled, about 3-4 minutes.
6. Serve warm.

Nutrition Info per Serving:
- Calories: 150
- Protein: 20g
- Carbohydrates: 7g
- Dietary Fiber: 2g
- Sugars: 4g
- Fat: 5g
- Saturated Fat: 1g
- Sodium: 200mg

Servings: 2
Cooking Time: 10 minutes

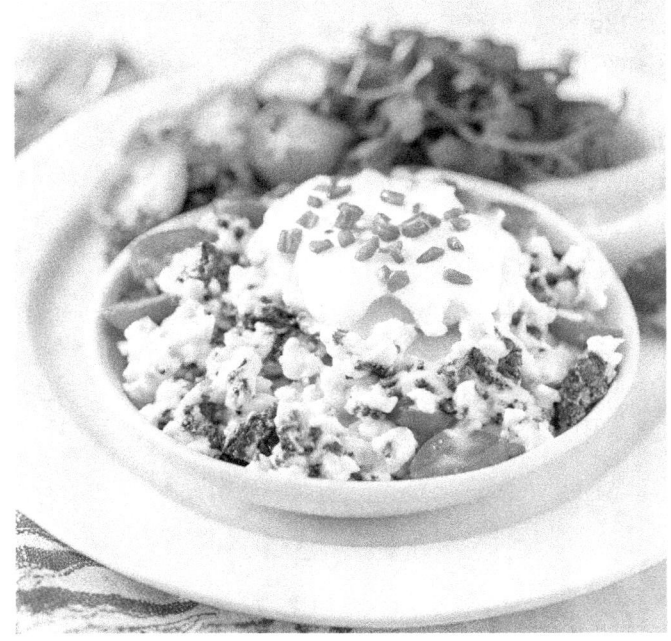

4. Avocado Toast on Whole Grain Bread

Ingredients:
- 2 slices whole grain bread
- 1 ripe avocado
- 1 tsp lemon juice
- 1/2 tsp ground black pepper
- 1/2 tsp garlic powder
- 1 tbsp chopped fresh cilantro (optional)

Instructions:
1. Toast the slices of whole grain bread until golden brown.
2. In a small bowl, mash the avocado with a fork. Add the lemon juice, black pepper, and garlic powder, mixing until smooth.
3. Spread the avocado mixture evenly on the toasted bread.
4. Top with chopped fresh cilantro if desired.
5. Serve immediately.

Nutrition Info per Serving:
- Calories: 250
- Protein: 6g
- Carbohydrates: 32g
- Dietary Fiber: 10g
- Sugars: 4g
- Fat: 12g
- Saturated Fat: 2g
- Sodium: 220mg

Servings: 1
Cooking Time: 5 minutes

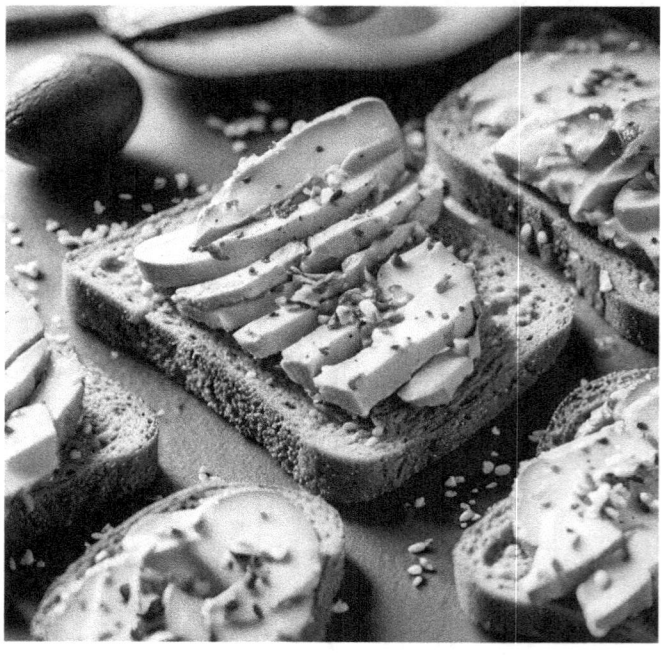

5. Peaches and Cream Smoothie

Ingredients:
- 1 cup unsweetened almond milk
- 1 cup frozen peach slices
- 1/2 cup Greek yogurt (fat-free)
- 1 tbsp honey (optional)
- 1 tsp vanilla extract
- 1 tbsp chia seeds

Instructions:
1. In a blender, combine the almond milk, frozen peach slices, Greek yogurt, honey, vanilla extract, and chia seeds.
2. Blend until smooth.
3. Pour into a glass and serve immediately.

Nutrition Info per Serving:
- Calories: 180
- Protein: 10g
- Carbohydrates: 30g
- Dietary Fiber: 5g
- Sugars: 20g
- Fat: 3g
- Saturated Fat: 0.5g
- Sodium: 90mg

Servings: 1
Cooking Time: 5 minutes

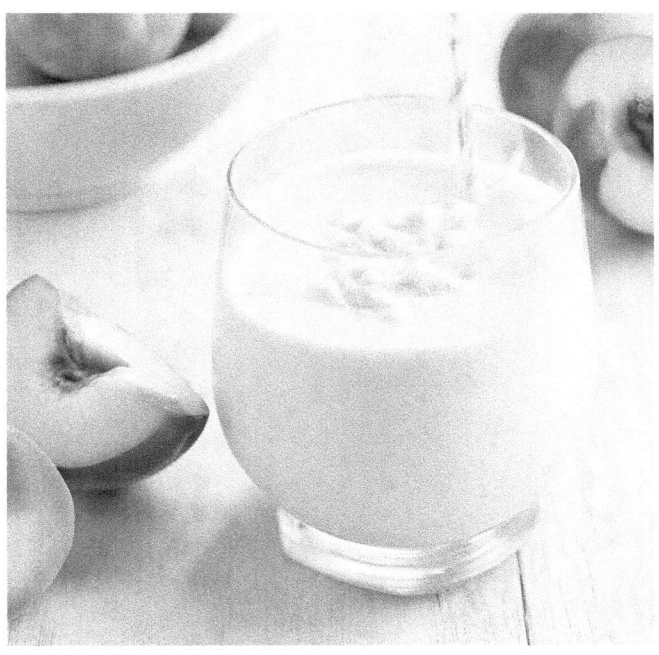

6. Carrot and Ginger Juice

Ingredients:
- 4 large carrots, peeled and chopped
- 1-inch piece of fresh ginger, peeled
- 1 apple, cored and chopped
- 1 cup cold water
- 1 tbsp lemon juice

Instructions:
1. In a blender, combine the carrots, ginger, apple, and cold water. Blend until smooth.
2. Strain the juice through a fine-mesh sieve or cheesecloth into a pitcher, pressing down to extract as much liquid as possible.
3. Stir in the lemon juice.
4. Serve chilled.

Nutrition Info per Serving:
- Calories: 80
- Protein: 1g
- Carbohydrates: 20g
- Dietary Fiber: 4g
- Sugars: 12g
- Fat: 0g
- Saturated Fat: 0g
- Sodium: 50mg

Servings: 2
Cooking Time: 10 minutes

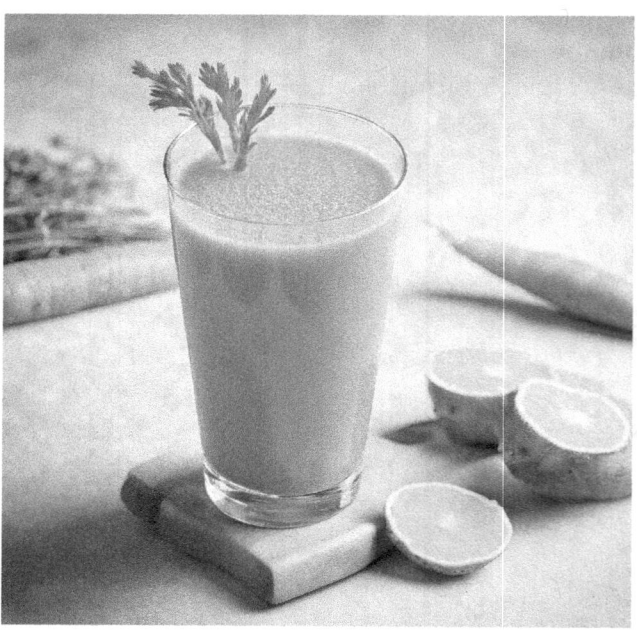

7. Papaya Salad

Ingredients:
- 1 ripe papaya, peeled, seeded, and cubed
- 1 cup cucumber, peeled and sliced
- 1/4 cup red onion, thinly sliced
- 1 tbsp fresh lime juice
- 1 tbsp chopped fresh mint leaves
- 1 tbsp chopped fresh cilantro

Instructions:
1. In a large bowl, combine the papaya, cucumber, and red onion.
2. Drizzle with lime juice and toss gently to combine.
3. Sprinkle with chopped mint and cilantro.
4. Serve immediately.

Nutrition Info per Serving:
- Calories: 90
- Protein: 1g
- Carbohydrates: 24g
- Dietary Fiber: 4g
- Sugars: 18g
- Fat: 0g
- Saturated Fat: 0g
- Sodium: 10mg

Servings: 2
Cooking Time: 10 minutes

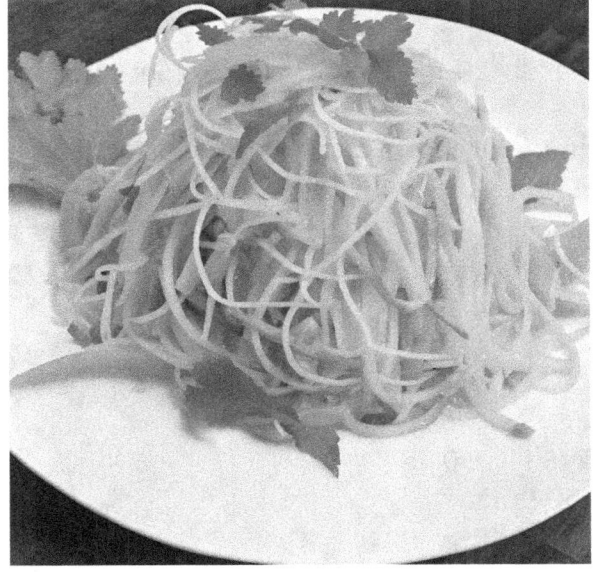

8. Oat Bran Muffins

Ingredients:
- 1 cup oat bran
- 1/2 cup whole wheat flour
- 1 tsp baking powder
- 1/2 tsp baking soda
- 1 tsp ground cinnamon
- 1/4 cup unsweetened applesauce
- 1/2 cup skim milk
- 1/4 cup honey
- 1 large egg white
- 1 tsp vanilla extract
- 1/2 cup fresh blueberries

Instructions:
1. Preheat the oven to 375°F (190°C). Line a muffin tin with paper liners.
2. In a large bowl, combine the oat bran, whole wheat flour, baking powder, baking soda, and cinnamon.
3. In another bowl, mix together the applesauce, skim milk, honey, egg white, and vanilla extract.
4. Pour the wet ingredients into the dry ingredients and stir until just combined.
5. Gently fold in the blueberries.
6. Divide the batter evenly among the muffin cups.
7. Bake for 18-20 minutes or until a toothpick inserted into the center comes out clean.
8. Cool in the pan for 5 minutes, then transfer to a wire rack to cool completely.

Nutrition Info per Serving:
- Calories: 130
- Protein: 4g
- Carbohydrates: 28g
- Dietary Fiber: 4g
- Sugars: 12g
- Fat: 1.5g
- Saturated Fat: 0.5g
- Sodium: 110mg

Servings: 8 muffins
Cooking Time: 25 minutes

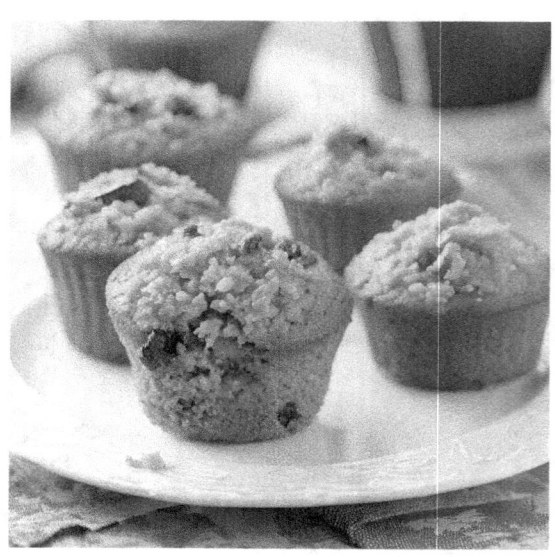

9. Buckwheat Pancakes

Ingredients:
- 1 cup buckwheat flour
- 1 tsp baking powder
- 1/2 tsp baking soda
- 1/2 tsp ground cinnamon
- 1 tbsp honey
- 1 cup skim milk
- 1 large egg white
- 1 tsp vanilla extract
- 1 tbsp olive oil (for cooking)

Instructions:
1. In a large bowl, whisk together the buckwheat flour, baking powder, baking soda, and cinnamon.
2. In another bowl, combine the honey, skim milk, egg white, and vanilla extract.
3. Pour the wet ingredients into the dry ingredients and stir until just combined.
4. Heat a non-stick skillet over medium heat and lightly brush with olive oil.
5. Pour 1/4 cup of batter onto the skillet for each pancake.
6. Cook until bubbles form on the surface and the edges look set, about 2-3 minutes.
7. Flip and cook for another 1-2 minutes until golden brown.
8. Serve warm with fresh fruit or a drizzle of honey.

Nutrition Info per Serving:
- Calories: 110
- Protein: 4g
- Carbohydrates: 20g
- Dietary Fiber: 3g
- Sugars: 6g
- Fat: 2g
- Saturated Fat: 0.5g
- Sodium: 150mg

Servings: 4 pancakes
Cooking Time: 15 minutes

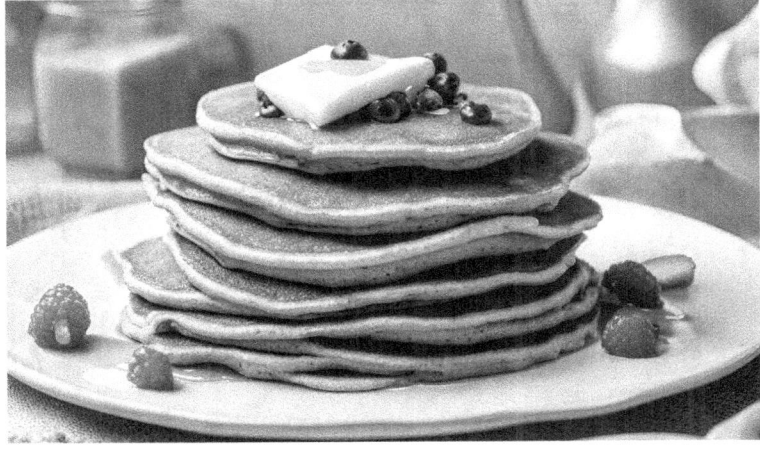

10. Vegetable Soup

Ingredients:
- 1 tbsp olive oil
- 1 onion, chopped
- 2 carrots, sliced
- 2 celery stalks, sliced
- 2 cloves garlic, minced
- 1 zucchini, chopped
- 1 cup green beans, trimmed and cut into 1-inch pieces
- 4 cups low-sodium vegetable broth
- 1 can (14.5 oz) diced tomatoes, no salt added
- 1 tsp dried basil
- 1 tsp dried oregano
- 1/2 tsp ground black pepper
- 2 cups spinach, chopped

Instructions:
1. Heat the olive oil in a large pot over medium heat.
2. Add the onion, carrots, and celery. Cook, stirring occasionally, until the vegetables are tender, about 5-7 minutes.
3. Add the garlic and cook for another minute until fragrant.
4. Stir in the zucchini and green beans, and cook for 3-4 minutes.
5. Add the vegetable broth, diced tomatoes, basil, oregano, and black pepper. Bring to a boil.
6. Reduce the heat and simmer for 20 minutes.
7. Stir in the spinach and cook until wilted, about 2 minutes.
8. Serve hot.

Nutrition Info per Serving:
- Calories: 90
- Protein: 3g
- Carbohydrates: 16g
- Dietary Fiber: 4g
- Sugars: 6g
- Fat: 3g
- Saturated Fat: 0.5g
- Sodium: 150mg

Servings: 4
Cooking Time: 35 minutes

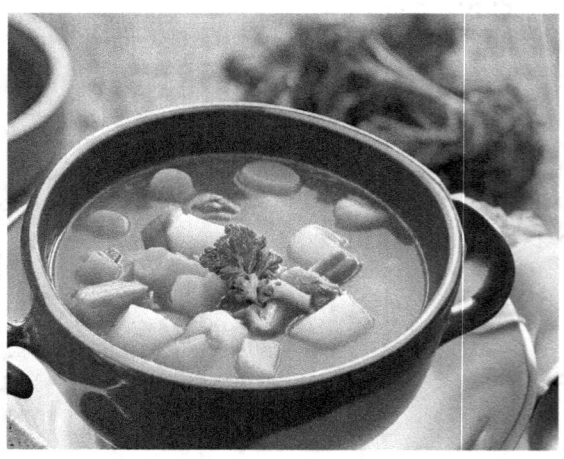

11. Barley Porridge

Ingredients:
- 1 cup barley
- 4 cups water or skim milk
- 1 apple, peeled and diced
- 1 tsp ground cinnamon
- 1 tbsp honey (optional)
- Fresh berries for topping (optional)

Instructions:
1. Rinse the barley under cold water.
2. In a medium saucepan, bring the water or skim milk to a boil.
3. Add the barley, reduce the heat to low, and simmer for about 45 minutes until the barley is tender and the liquid is absorbed.
4. Stir in the diced apple, ground cinnamon, and honey.
5. Serve warm, topped with fresh berries if desired.

Nutrition Info per Serving:
- Calories: 180
- Protein: 5g
- Carbohydrates: 39g
- Dietary Fiber: 7g
- Sugars: 12g
- Fat: 1g
- Saturated Fat: 0g
- Sodium: 10mg

Servings: 4
Cooking Time: 50 minutes

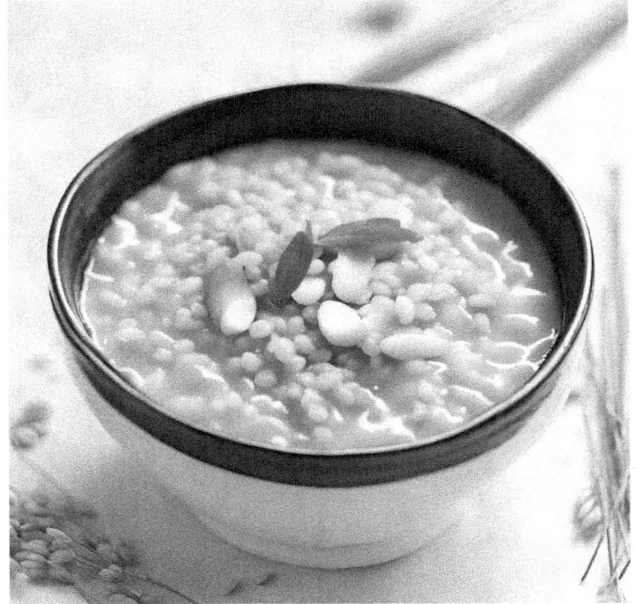

12. Cucumber Tomato Sandwich

Ingredients:
- 4 slices whole grain bread
- 1 cucumber, thinly sliced
- 2 tomatoes, thinly sliced
- 1/4 cup hummus
- 1 tbsp fresh basil leaves, chopped
- 1 tbsp fresh mint leaves, chopped

Instructions:
1. Toast the slices of whole grain bread until golden brown.
2. Spread hummus evenly on each slice of toast.
3. Arrange cucumber and tomato slices on two pieces of toast.
4. Sprinkle with chopped basil and mint.
5. Top with the remaining slices of toast to make sandwiches.
6. Serve immediately.

Nutrition Info per Serving:
- Calories: 220
- Protein: 7g
- Carbohydrates: 38g
- Dietary Fiber: 8g
- Sugars: 6g
- Fat: 6g
- Saturated Fat: 1g
- Sodium: 200mg

Servings: 2
Cooking Time: 10 minutes

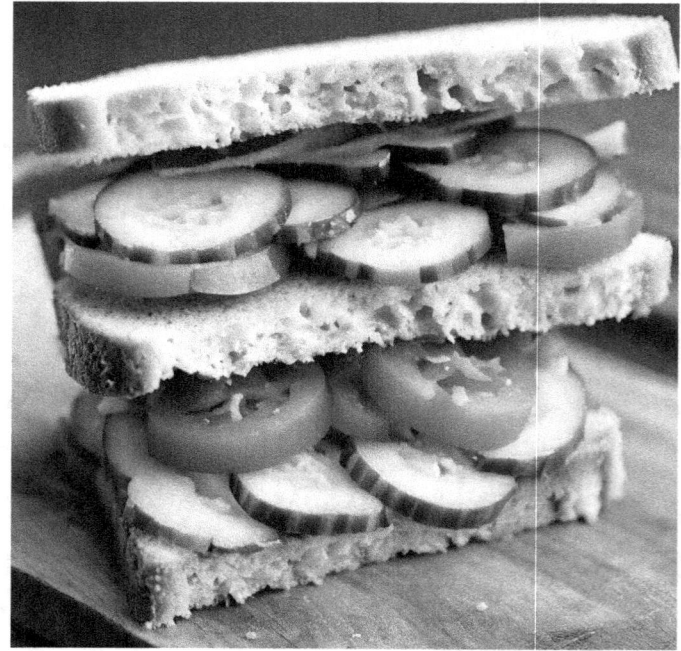

13. Chia Seed Pudding

Ingredients:
- 1/4 cup chia seeds
- 1 cup unsweetened almond milk
- 1 tbsp honey
- 1/2 tsp vanilla extract
- Fresh fruit (e.g., berries, mango) for topping

Instructions:
1. In a medium bowl, whisk together the chia seeds, almond milk, honey, and vanilla extract.
2. Cover and refrigerate for at least 4 hours, or overnight, until the mixture thickens to a pudding-like consistency.
3. Stir the pudding to ensure even distribution of chia seeds.
4. Serve topped with fresh fruit.

Nutrition Info per Serving:
- Calories: 150
- Protein: 4g
- Carbohydrates: 18g
- Dietary Fiber: 10g
- Sugars: 10g
- Fat: 7g
- Saturated Fat: 0.5g
- Sodium: 60mg

Servings: 2
Cooking Time: 5 minutes (plus 4 hours chilling time)

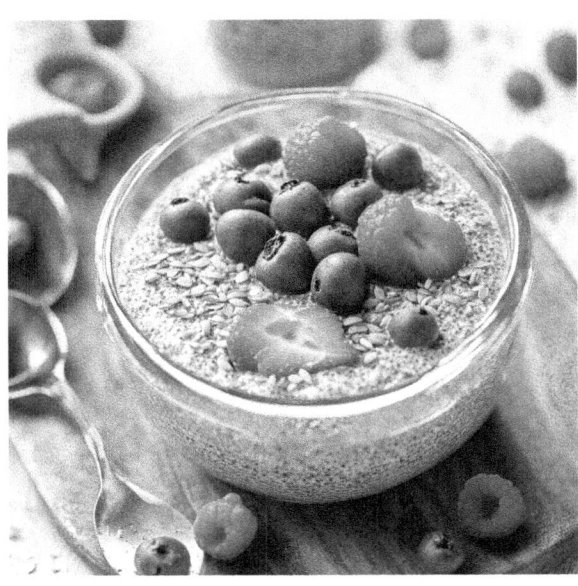

14. Vegetable Omelette

Ingredients:
- 4 egg whites
- 1/4 cup skim milk
- 1/2 cup bell pepper, diced
- 1/2 cup mushrooms, sliced
- 1/4 cup onion, finely chopped
- 1/2 cup spinach, chopped
- 1 tbsp olive oil
- 1/2 tsp ground black pepper

Instructions:
1. In a medium bowl, whisk together the egg whites, skim milk, and black pepper.
2. Heat the olive oil in a non-stick skillet over medium heat.
3. Add the onion and bell pepper, and sauté for 2-3 minutes until softened.
4. Add the mushrooms and cook for another 2 minutes.
5. Stir in the spinach and cook until wilted, about 1 minute.
6. Pour the egg mixture into the skillet, swirling to coat the vegetables evenly.
7. Cook until the eggs are set, about 3-4 minutes, then fold the omelette in half.
8. Serve warm.

Nutrition Info per Serving:
- Calories: 120
- Protein: 14g
- Carbohydrates: 6g
- Dietary Fiber: 2g
- Sugars: 4g
- Fat: 4g
- Saturated Fat: 0.5g
- Sodium: 150mg

Servings: 2
Cooking Time: 10 minutes

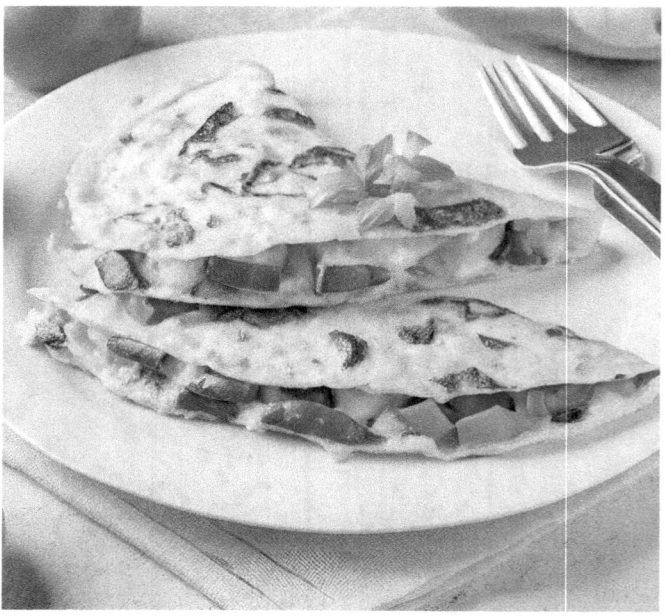

15. Berry Fruit Salad

Ingredients:
- 1 cup strawberries, hulled and sliced
- 1 cup blueberries
- 1 cup raspberries
- 1 cup blackberries
- 2 tbsp fresh mint leaves, chopped
- 1 tbsp honey (optional)
- 1 tbsp fresh lemon juice

Instructions:
1. In a large bowl, combine the strawberries, blueberries, raspberries, and blackberries.
2. Add the chopped mint leaves and toss gently to combine.
3. Drizzle with honey and lemon juice, and toss again.
4. Serve immediately.

Nutrition Info per Serving:
- Calories: 90
- Protein: 1g
- Carbohydrates: 22g
- Dietary Fiber: 8g
- Sugars: 12g
- Fat: 1g
- Saturated Fat: 0g
- Sodium: 5mg

Servings: 4
Cooking Time: 5 minutes

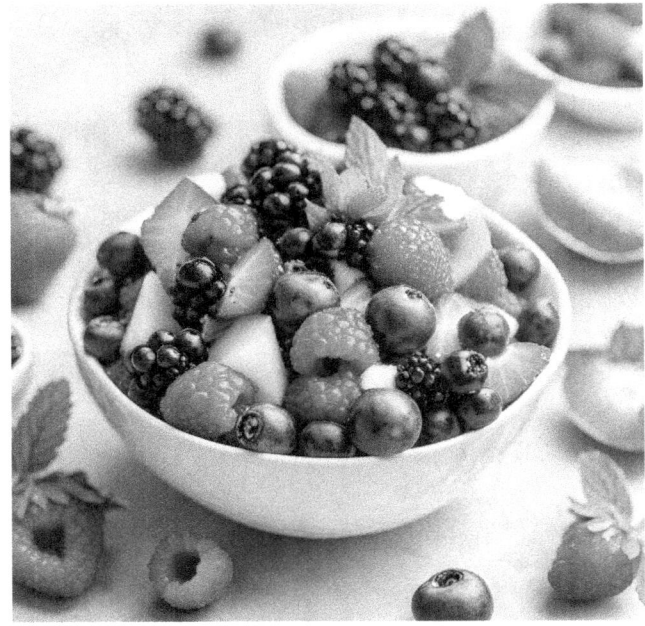

16. Pumpkin Soup

Ingredients:
- 1 tbsp olive oil
- 1 onion, chopped
- 2 cloves garlic, minced
- 4 cups pumpkin, peeled and cubed
- 4 cups low-sodium vegetable broth
- 1/2 tsp ground black pepper
- 1/2 tsp ground nutmeg
- 1/2 cup skim milk
- Fresh parsley for garnish

Instructions:
1. Heat the olive oil in a large pot over medium heat.
2. Add the onion and cook until softened, about 5 minutes.
3. Add the garlic and cook for another minute.
4. Stir in the pumpkin, vegetable broth, black pepper, and nutmeg.
5. Bring to a boil, then reduce the heat and simmer until the pumpkin is tender, about 20 minutes.
6. Use an immersion blender to puree the soup until smooth (or transfer to a blender in batches).
7. Stir in the skim milk and heat through without boiling.
8. Serve warm, garnished with fresh parsley.

Nutrition Info per Serving:
- Calories: 100
- Protein: 3g
- Carbohydrates: 20g
- Dietary Fiber: 4g
- Sugars: 8g
- Fat: 3g
- Saturated Fat: 0.5g
- Sodium: 150mg

Servings: 4
Cooking Time: 30 minutes

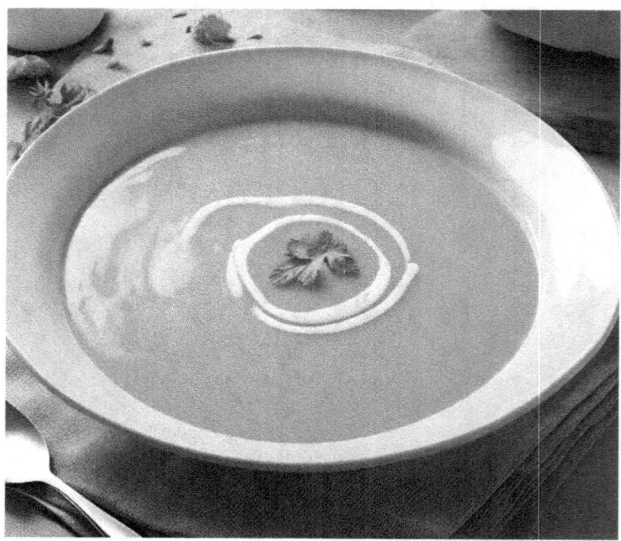

17. Mango Smoothie

Ingredients:
- 1 cup fresh or frozen mango chunks
- 1/2 cup plain Greek yogurt (fat-free)
- 1/2 cup unsweetened almond milk
- 1 tbsp chia seeds
- 1 tbsp honey (optional)
- 1/2 tsp vanilla extract

Instructions:
1. In a blender, combine the mango chunks, Greek yogurt, almond milk, chia seeds, honey, and vanilla extract.
2. Blend until smooth.
3. Pour into a glass and serve immediately.

Nutrition Info per Serving:
- Calories: 180
- Protein: 8g
- Carbohydrates: 32g
- Dietary Fiber: 5g
- Sugars: 24g
- Fat: 3g
- Saturated Fat: 0g
- Sodium: 70mg

Servings: 1
Cooking Time: 5 minutes

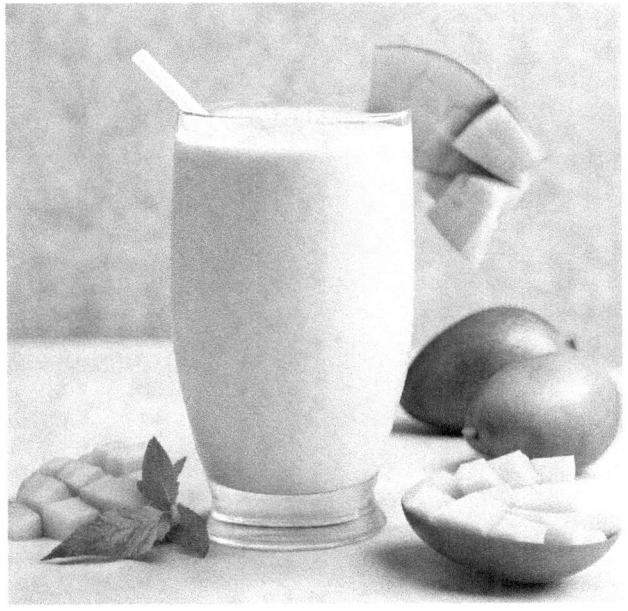

18. Sautéed Vegetables

Ingredients:
- 1 tbsp olive oil
- 1 cup bell pepper, sliced
- 1 cup zucchini, sliced
- 1 cup mushrooms, sliced
- 1/2 cup onion, thinly sliced
- 1 tsp dried oregano
- 1 tsp garlic powder

Instructions:
1. Heat the olive oil in a large skillet over medium heat.
2. Add the onion and bell pepper, and sauté for 3-4 minutes until softened.
3. Add the zucchini and mushrooms, and continue to cook for another 5-6 minutes until all the vegetables are tender.
4. Sprinkle with dried oregano and garlic powder, and stir well.
5. Serve warm.

Nutrition Info per Serving:
- Calories: 100
- Protein: 2g
- Carbohydrates: 10g
- Dietary Fiber: 3g
- Sugars: 5g
- Fat: 7g
- Saturated Fat: 1g
- Sodium: 10mg

Servings: 2
Cooking Time: 10 minutes

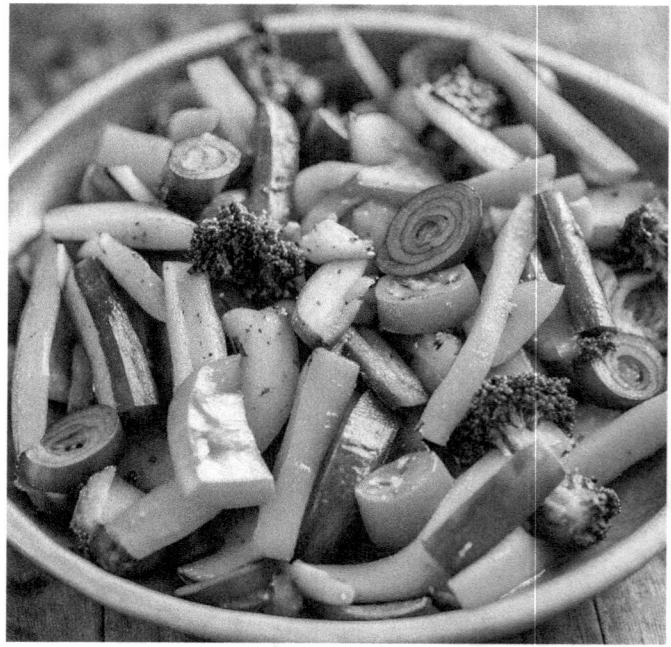

19. Almond Milk Porridge

Ingredients:
- 1 cup rolled oats
- 2 cups unsweetened almond milk
- 1 ripe banana, mashed
- 1 tsp ground cinnamon
- 1 tsp vanilla extract
- 1 tbsp flaxseeds
- Fresh berries for topping (optional)

Instructions:
1. In a medium saucepan, bring the almond milk to a boil.
2. Add the rolled oats and reduce the heat to a simmer. Cook for about 5 minutes, stirring occasionally.
3. Stir in the mashed banana, ground cinnamon, vanilla extract, and flaxseeds. Continue to cook for another 2-3 minutes until the oats are creamy.
4. Remove from heat and let sit for a minute.
5. Serve warm, topped with fresh berries if desired.

Nutrition Info per Serving:
- Calories: 220
- Protein: 5g
- Carbohydrates: 40g
- Dietary Fiber: 8g
- Sugars: 10g
- Fat: 5g
- Saturated Fat: 0g
- Sodium: 30mg

Servings: 2
Cooking Time: 10 minutes

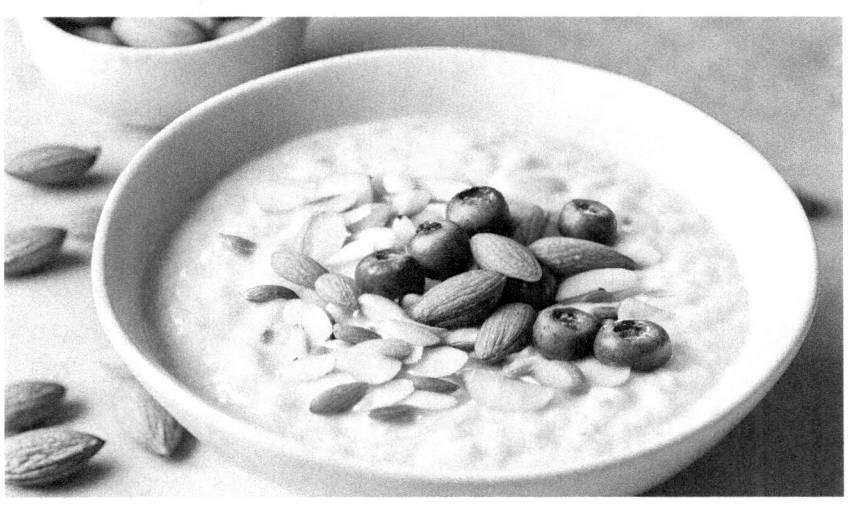

20. Spelt Toast with Banana

Ingredients:
- 2 slices spelt bread
- 1 ripe banana, sliced
- 1 tbsp almond butter
- 1/2 tsp ground cinnamon

Instructions:
1. Toast the slices of spelt bread until golden brown.
2. Spread almond butter evenly on each slice of toast.
3. Arrange banana slices on top of the almond butter.
4. Sprinkle with ground cinnamon.
5. Serve immediately.

Nutrition Info per Serving:
- Calories: 250
- Protein: 6g
- Carbohydrates: 40g
- Dietary Fiber: 6g
- Sugars: 12g
- Fat: 8g
- Saturated Fat: 1g
- Sodium: 150mg

Servings: 1
Cooking Time: 5 minutes

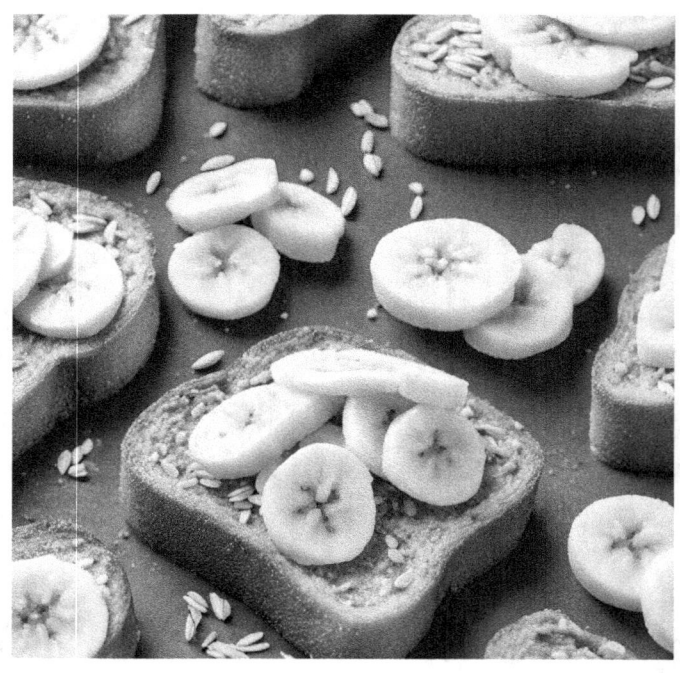

21. Boiled Potatoes with Dill

Ingredients:
- 4 medium potatoes, peeled and cubed
- 1 tbsp olive oil
- 2 tbsp fresh dill, chopped
- 1/2 tsp garlic powder
- 1/2 tsp ground black pepper

Instructions:
1. In a large pot, bring water to a boil. Add the cubed potatoes and cook for about 15-20 minutes, or until tender.
2. Drain the potatoes and transfer them to a large bowl.
3. Drizzle the olive oil over the potatoes and sprinkle with garlic powder and ground black pepper.
4. Gently toss to coat the potatoes evenly.
5. Garnish with fresh dill and serve warm.

Nutrition Info per Serving:
- Calories: 160
- Protein: 3g
- Carbohydrates: 30g
- Dietary Fiber: 4g
- Sugars: 2g
- Fat: 4g
- Saturated Fat: 0.5g
- Sodium: 20mg

Servings: 4
Cooking Time: 20 minutes

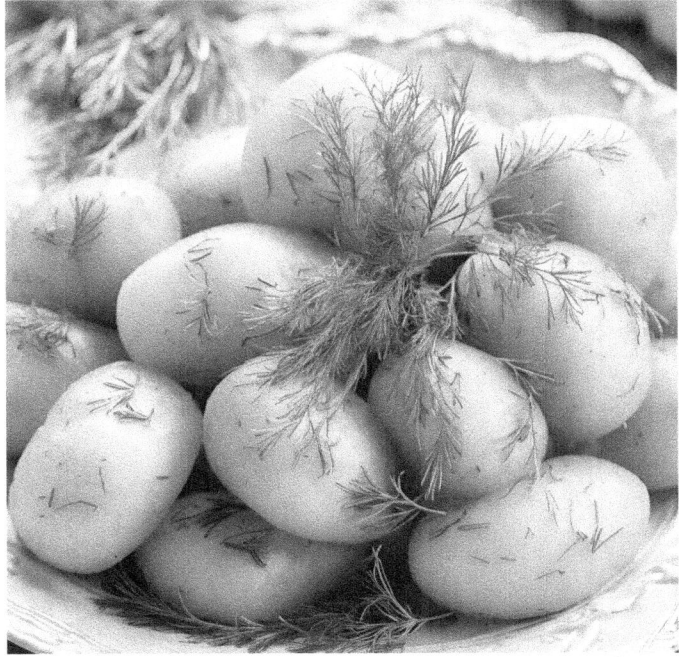

22. Buckwheat Crepes

Ingredients:
- 1 cup buckwheat flour
- 1 cup skim milk
- 2 large egg whites
- 1 tbsp olive oil (for cooking)
- 1 tsp vanilla extract
- 1 tbsp honey (optional)

Instructions:
1. In a medium bowl, whisk together the buckwheat flour, skim milk, egg whites, vanilla extract, and honey until smooth.
2. Heat a non-stick skillet over medium heat and lightly brush with olive oil.
3. Pour about 1/4 cup of batter into the skillet and swirl to spread evenly.
4. Cook for 2-3 minutes until the edges start to lift and the bottom is lightly browned. Flip and cook for another 1-2 minutes.
5. Repeat with the remaining batter.
6. Serve warm with fresh fruit or a drizzle of honey if desired.

Nutrition Info per Serving:
- Calories: 100
- Protein: 5g
- Carbohydrates: 18g
- Dietary Fiber: 2g
- Sugars: 4g
- Fat: 2g
- Saturated Fat: 0.5g
- Sodium: 30mg

Servings: 4 crepes
Cooking Time: 15 minutes

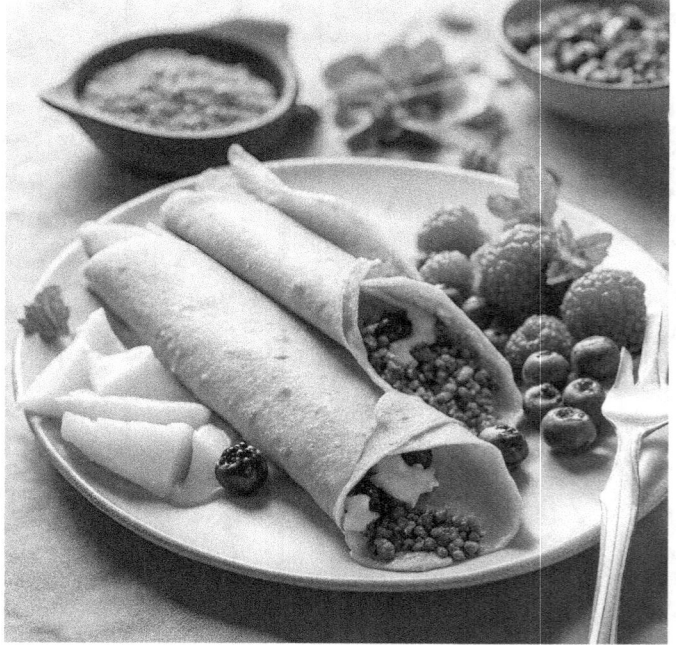

23. Rice and Pea Salad

Ingredients:
- 1 cup cooked brown rice (cooled)
- 1 cup green peas (fresh or frozen)
- 1/2 cup red bell pepper, diced
- 1/4 cup red onion, finely chopped
- 2 tbsp fresh parsley, chopped
- 1 tbsp olive oil
- 1 tbsp lemon juice
- 1/2 tsp ground black pepper

Instructions:
1. If using frozen peas, blanch them in boiling water for 2-3 minutes until tender, then drain and cool.
2. In a large bowl, combine the cooked brown rice, green peas, red bell pepper, red onion, and fresh parsley.
3. In a small bowl, whisk together the olive oil, lemon juice, and ground black pepper.
4. Pour the dressing over the rice mixture and toss gently to combine.
5. Serve chilled or at room temperature.

Nutrition Info per Serving:
- Calories: 180
- Protein: 5g
- Carbohydrates: 28g
- Dietary Fiber: 4g
- Sugars: 3g
- Fat: 6g
- Saturated Fat: 0.5g
- Sodium: 10mg

Servings: 4
Cooking Time: 15 minutes

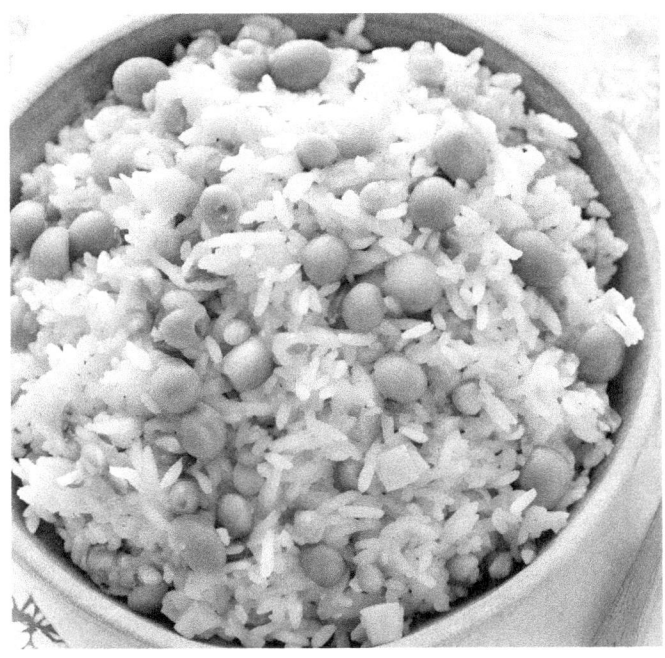

Poultry Recipes

1. Herb-Roasted Turkey Breast
Ingredients:
- 1 (2-3 lb) boneless turkey breast
- 2 tbsp olive oil
- 1 tbsp fresh rosemary, chopped
- 1 tbsp fresh thyme, chopped
- 1 tbsp fresh sage, chopped
- 2 cloves garlic, minced
- 1/2 tsp ground black pepper
- 1 lemon, sliced

Instructions:
1. Preheat the oven to 350°F (175°C).
2. In a small bowl, mix together the olive oil, rosemary, thyme, sage, garlic, and ground black pepper.
3. Rub the herb mixture all over the turkey breast.
4. Place the lemon slices on the bottom of a roasting pan and place the turkey breast on top of the lemons.
5. Roast in the preheated oven for 1.5 to 2 hours, or until the internal temperature reaches 165°F (74°C).
6. Let the turkey rest for 10 minutes before slicing.
7. Serve warm.

Nutrition Info per Serving:
- Calories: 180
- Protein: 30g
- Carbohydrates: 1g
- Dietary Fiber: 0g
- Sugars: 0g
- Fat: 6g
- Saturated Fat: 1g
- Sodium: 70mg

Servings: 6
Cooking Time: 2 hours

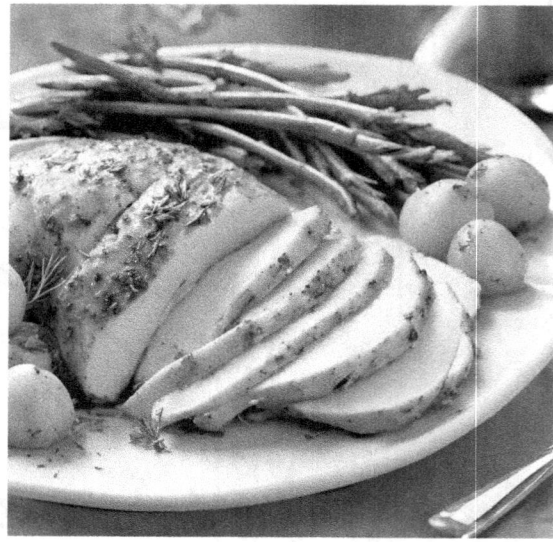

2. Chicken and Vegetable Soup

Ingredients:
- 1 tbsp olive oil
- 1 onion, chopped
- 2 carrots, sliced
- 2 celery stalks, sliced
- 2 cloves garlic, minced
- 1 zucchini, chopped
- 1 cup green beans, trimmed and cut into 1-inch pieces
- 4 cups low-sodium chicken broth
- 1 cup cooked chicken breast, shredded
- 1/2 tsp dried thyme
- 1/2 tsp dried oregano
- 1/2 tsp ground black pepper
- 2 cups spinach, chopped

Instructions:
1. Heat the olive oil in a large pot over medium heat.
2. Add the onion, carrots, and celery. Cook, stirring occasionally, until the vegetables are tender, about 5-7 minutes.
3. Add the garlic and cook for another minute until fragrant.
4. Stir in the zucchini and green beans, and cook for 3-4 minutes.
5. Add the chicken broth, shredded chicken, thyme, oregano, and black pepper. Bring to a boil.
6. Reduce the heat and simmer for 20 minutes.
7. Stir in the spinach and cook until wilted, about 2 minutes.
8. Serve hot.

Nutrition Info per Serving:
- Calories: 150
- Protein: 15g
- Carbohydrates: 10g
- Dietary Fiber: 3g
- Sugars: 4g
- Fat: 5g
- Saturated Fat: 1g
- Sodium: 150mg

Servings: 4
Cooking Time: 35 minutes

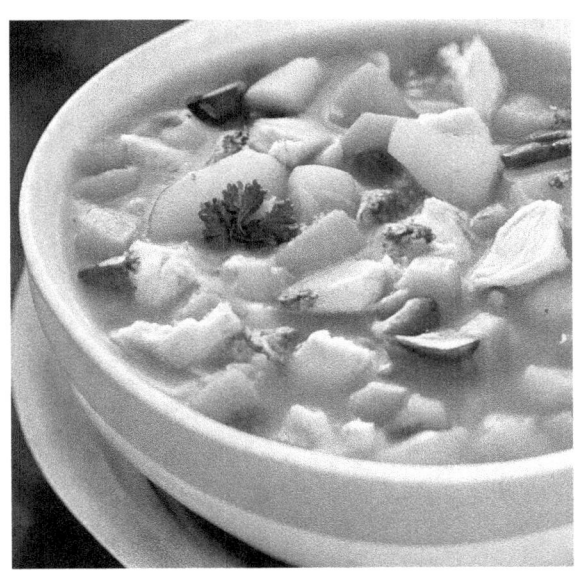

3. Ginger Chicken Stir-Fry

Ingredients:
- 1 lb chicken breast, sliced into thin strips
- 1 tbsp olive oil
- 1-inch piece fresh ginger, grated
- 2 cloves garlic, minced
- 1 red bell pepper, sliced
- 1 yellow bell pepper, sliced
- 1 cup snow peas
- 1 cup broccoli florets
- 2 tbsp low-sodium soy sauce
- 1 tbsp honey
- 1 tbsp cornstarch mixed with 2 tbsp water

Instructions:
1. Heat the olive oil in a large skillet or wok over medium-high heat.
2. Add the ginger and garlic, and stir-fry for 1 minute until fragrant.
3. Add the chicken strips and cook until no longer pink, about 5-7 minutes.
4. Add the bell peppers, snow peas, and broccoli, and stir-fry for another 5 minutes until the vegetables are tender-crisp.
5. Stir in the soy sauce and honey, and cook for 2 minutes.
6. Add the cornstarch mixture and cook for another minute until the sauce thickens.
7. Serve hot.

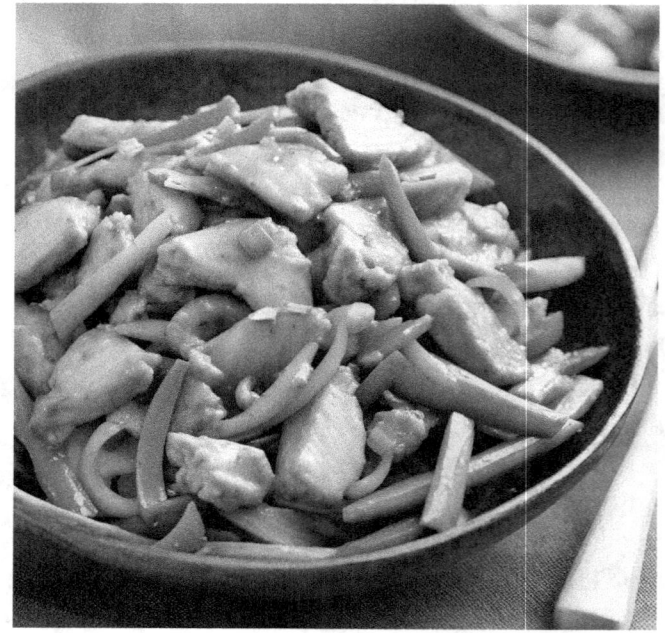

Nutrition Info per Serving:
- Calories: 220
- Protein: 28g
- Carbohydrates: 15g
- Dietary Fiber: 4g
- Sugars: 8g
- Fat: 7g
- Saturated Fat: 1g
- Sodium: 200mg

Servings: 4
Cooking Time: 20 minutes

4. Lemon Garlic Chicken

Ingredients:
- 4 boneless, skinless chicken breasts
- 2 tbsp olive oil
- 4 cloves garlic, minced
- 1 lemon, juiced and zested
- 1 tbsp fresh parsley, chopped
- 1/2 tsp ground black pepper

Instructions:
1. Preheat the oven to 375°F (190°C).
2. In a small bowl, mix together the olive oil, garlic, lemon juice, lemon zest, parsley, and ground black pepper.
3. Place the chicken breasts in a baking dish and pour the lemon-garlic mixture over them, coating each breast evenly.
4. Bake in the preheated oven for 25-30 minutes, or until the chicken is cooked through and the internal temperature reaches 165°F (74°C).
5. Let the chicken rest for 5 minutes before serving.
6. Serve warm.

Nutrition Info per Serving:
- Calories: 200
- Protein: 28g
- Carbohydrates: 2g
- Dietary Fiber: 0g
- Sugars: 0g
- Fat: 8g
- Saturated Fat: 1.5g
- Sodium: 70mg

Servings: 4
Cooking Time: 30 minutes

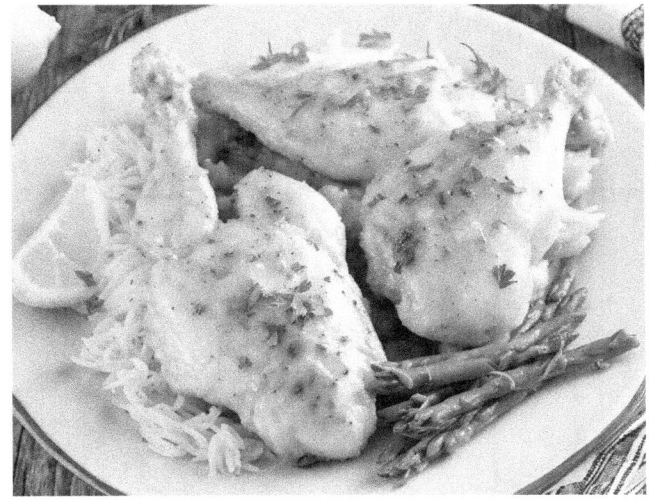

5. Turkey Meatballs

Ingredients:
- 1 lb ground turkey (lean)
- 1/4 cup whole wheat breadcrumbs
- 1/4 cup grated Parmesan cheese
- 1 large egg white
- 2 cloves garlic, minced
- 1 tbsp fresh parsley, chopped
- 1/2 tsp dried oregano
- 1/2 tsp ground black pepper

Instructions:
1. Preheat the oven to 375°F (190°C). Line a baking sheet with parchment paper.
2. In a large bowl, combine the ground turkey, breadcrumbs, Parmesan cheese, egg white, garlic, parsley, oregano, and black pepper. Mix until well combined.
3. Shape the mixture into 1-inch meatballs and place them on the prepared baking sheet.
4. Bake in the preheated oven for 20-25 minutes, or until the meatballs are cooked through and lightly browned.
5. Serve warm with your favorite sauce or as part of a meal.

Nutrition Info per Serving:
- Calories: 180
- Protein: 22g
- Carbohydrates: 6g
- Dietary Fiber: 1g
- Sugars: 0g
- Fat: 7g
- Saturated Fat: 2g
- Sodium: 150mg

Servings: 4
Cooking Time: 25 minutes

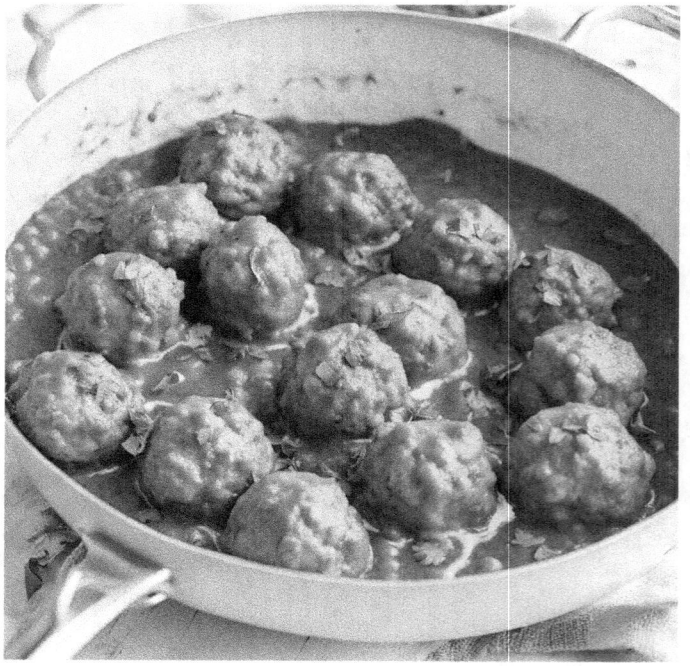

6. Chicken Congee

Ingredients:
- 1 cup jasmine rice
- 8 cups low-sodium chicken broth
- 1 boneless, skinless chicken breast
- 1-inch piece fresh ginger, sliced
- 2 cloves garlic, minced
- 2 green onions, chopped
- 1 tbsp low-sodium soy sauce
- 1/2 tsp ground black pepper

Instructions:
1. Rinse the jasmine rice under cold water until the water runs clear.
2. In a large pot, combine the rice, chicken broth, chicken breast, ginger, and garlic. Bring to a boil over medium-high heat.
3. Reduce the heat to low and simmer, stirring occasionally, until the rice is broken down and the congee is thick and creamy, about 1.5 to 2 hours.
4. Remove the chicken breast, shred it with two forks, and return it to the pot.
5. Stir in the soy sauce and ground black pepper.
6. Serve hot, garnished with chopped green onions.

Nutrition Info per Serving:
- Calories: 200
- Protein: 15g
- Carbohydrates: 25g
- Dietary Fiber: 1g
- Sugars: 0g
- Fat: 4g
- Saturated Fat: 1g
- Sodium: 250mg

Servings: 6
Cooking Time: 2 hours

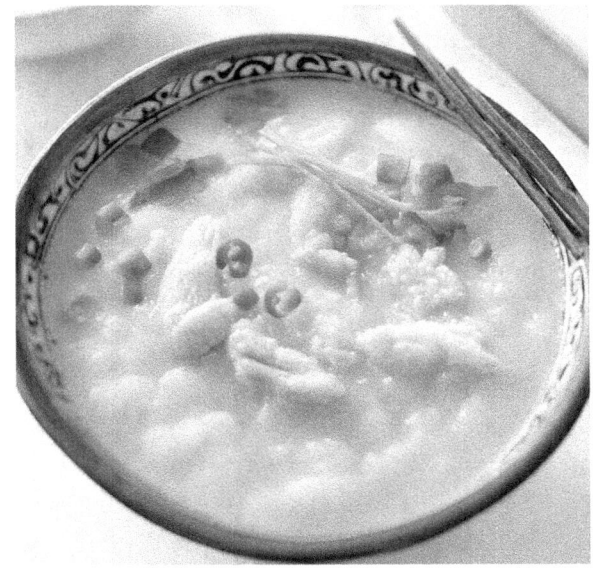

7. Poached Chicken Salad

Ingredients:
- 2 boneless, skinless chicken breasts
- 4 cups low-sodium chicken broth
- 1 bay leaf
- 1 tbsp olive oil
- 1 tbsp lemon juice
- 1/2 tsp ground black pepper
- 4 cups mixed greens (spinach, arugula, lettuce)
- 1/2 cup cherry tomatoes, halved
- 1/2 cucumber, sliced
- 1/4 cup red onion, thinly sliced

Instructions:
1. In a large pot, bring the chicken broth to a simmer. Add the chicken breasts and bay leaf.
2. Poach the chicken for 15-20 minutes, or until cooked through and no longer pink inside.
3. Remove the chicken from the broth and let cool. Once cool, shred the chicken into bite-sized pieces.
4. In a small bowl, whisk together the olive oil, lemon juice, and ground black pepper.
5. In a large bowl, combine the mixed greens, cherry tomatoes, cucumber, red onion, and shredded chicken.
6. Drizzle the dressing over the salad and toss gently to combine.
7. Serve immediately.

Nutrition Info per Serving:
- Calories: 220
- Protein: 25g
- Carbohydrates: 10g
- Dietary Fiber: 3g
- Sugars: 4g
- Fat: 10g
- Saturated Fat: 1.5g
- Sodium: 150mg

Servings: 4
Cooking Time: 25 minutes

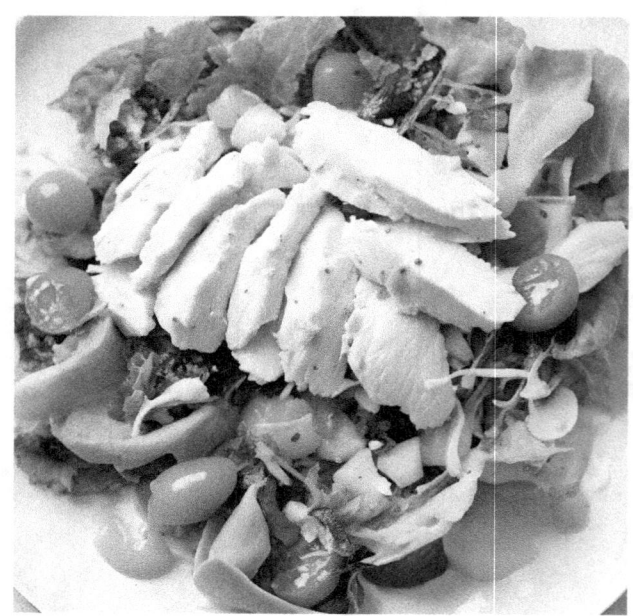

8. Smoked Turkey Wrap

Ingredients:
- 4 whole grain tortillas
- 8 oz smoked turkey breast, thinly sliced
- 1 avocado, sliced
- 1 cup spinach leaves
- 1/2 cup shredded carrots
- 1/2 cup cucumber, julienned
- 2 tbsp hummus
- 1 tbsp lemon juice

Instructions:
1. Spread 1/2 tbsp of hummus on each tortilla.
2. Layer with smoked turkey, avocado slices, spinach leaves, shredded carrots, and cucumber.
3. Drizzle with lemon juice.
4. Roll up each tortilla tightly and slice in half.
5. Serve immediately.

Nutrition Info per Serving:
- Calories: 300
- Protein: 20g
- Carbohydrates: 40g
- Dietary Fiber: 8g
- Sugars: 3g
- Fat: 10g
- Saturated Fat: 2g
- Sodium: 450mg

Servings: 4
Cooking Time: 10 minutes

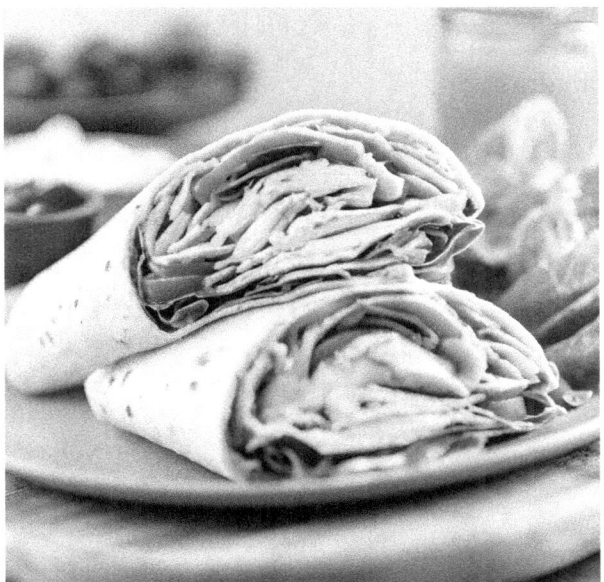

9. Balsamic Chicken

Ingredients:
- 4 boneless, skinless chicken breasts
- 1/4 cup balsamic vinegar
- 2 tbsp olive oil
- 2 cloves garlic, minced
- 1 tbsp fresh basil, chopped
- 1/2 tsp ground black pepper

Instructions:
1. Preheat the oven to 375°F (190°C).
2. In a small bowl, whisk together the balsamic vinegar, olive oil, garlic, basil, and ground black pepper.
3. Place the chicken breasts in a baking dish and pour the balsamic mixture over them, turning to coat evenly.
4. Bake in the preheated oven for 25-30 minutes, or until the chicken is cooked through and the internal temperature reaches 165°F (74°C).
5. Let the chicken rest for 5 minutes before serving.
6. Serve warm.

Nutrition Info per Serving:
- Calories: 200
- Protein: 28g
- Carbohydrates: 4g
- Dietary Fiber: 0g
- Sugars: 2g
- Fat: 8g
- Saturated Fat: 1.5g
- Sodium: 120mg

Servings: 4
Cooking Time: 30 minutes

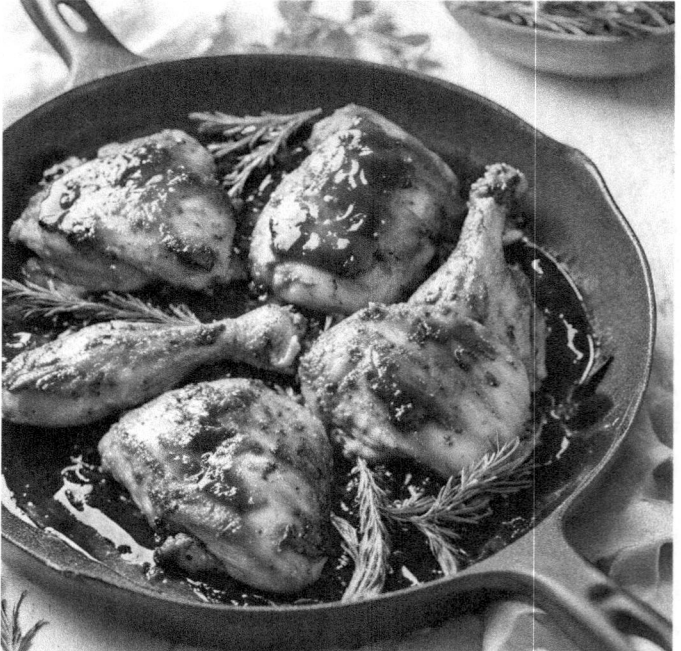

10. Turkey and Rice Pilaf

Ingredients:
- 1 lb ground turkey (lean)
- 1 tbsp olive oil
- 1 onion, chopped
- 1 carrot, grated
- 1 cup brown rice
- 2 cups low-sodium chicken broth
- 1/2 tsp ground black pepper
- 1/2 tsp dried thyme
- 1/2 cup peas (fresh or frozen)
- 1/4 cup fresh parsley, chopped

Instructions:
1. In a large skillet, heat the olive oil over medium heat.
2. Add the onion and cook until softened, about 3-4 minutes.
3. Add the ground turkey and cook until browned, about 5-7 minutes.
4. Stir in the grated carrot, brown rice, chicken broth, black pepper, and thyme.
5. Bring to a boil, then reduce heat to low, cover, and simmer for 45 minutes or until the rice is tender.
6. Stir in the peas and cook for an additional 5 minutes.
7. Remove from heat and stir in the fresh parsley.
8. Serve warm.

Nutrition Info per Serving:
- Calories: 300
- Protein: 20g
- Carbohydrates: 38g
- Dietary Fiber: 5g
- Sugars: 4g
- Fat: 9g
- Saturated Fat: 1.5g
- Sodium: 150mg

Servings: 4
Cooking Time: 55 minutes

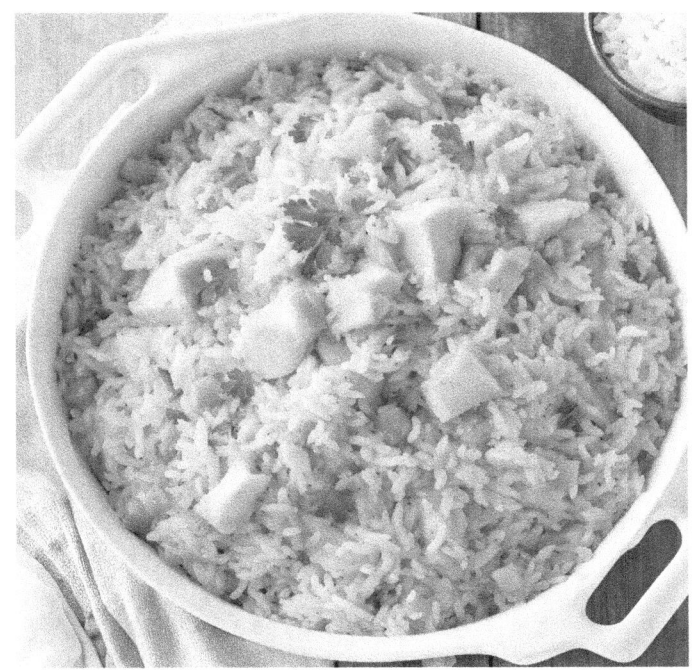

11. Chicken Vegetable Kabobs

Ingredients:
- 1 lb boneless, skinless chicken breasts, cut into 1-inch cubes
- 1 red bell pepper, cut into 1-inch pieces
- 1 yellow bell pepper, cut into 1-inch pieces
- 1 zucchini, sliced into rounds
- 1 red onion, cut into 1-inch pieces
- 2 tbsp olive oil
- 1 tbsp lemon juice
- 1 tsp dried oregano
- 1/2 tsp ground black pepper

Instructions:
1. In a large bowl, mix together the olive oil, lemon juice, oregano, and black pepper.
2. Add the chicken cubes and vegetables to the bowl, tossing to coat.
3. Thread the chicken and vegetables onto skewers, alternating pieces.
4. Preheat the grill to medium-high heat.
5. Grill the kabobs for 10-12 minutes, turning occasionally, until the chicken is cooked through and the vegetables are tender.
6. Serve warm.

Nutrition Info per Serving:
- Calories: 220
- Protein: 25g
- Carbohydrates: 10g
- Dietary Fiber: 3g
- Sugars: 4g
- Fat: 10g
- Saturated Fat: 1.5g
- Sodium: 100mg

Servings: 4
Cooking Time: 15 minute

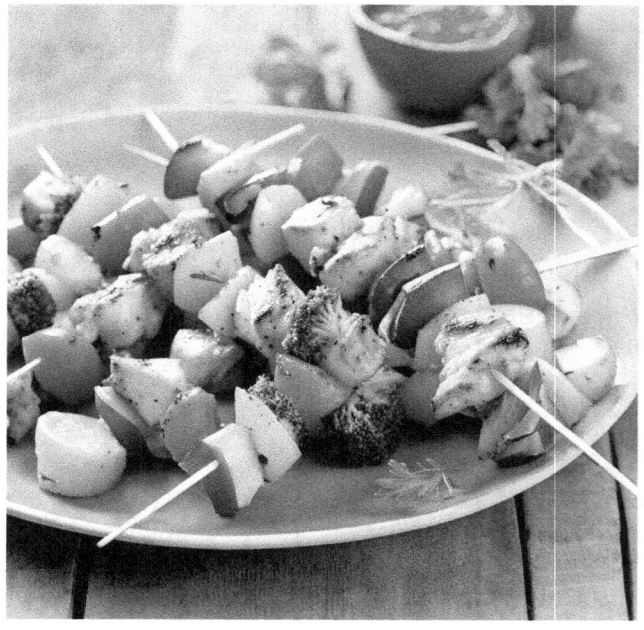

12. Orange-Glazed Chicken

Ingredients:
- 4 boneless, skinless chicken breasts
- 1/4 cup orange juice
- 2 tbsp honey
- 1 tbsp soy sauce (low sodium)
- 2 cloves garlic, minced
- 1/2 tsp ground ginger
- 1/2 tsp ground black pepper
- 1 tbsp olive oil

Instructions:
1. In a small bowl, whisk together the orange juice, honey, soy sauce, garlic, ginger, and black pepper.
2. Heat the olive oil in a large skillet over medium heat.
3. Add the chicken breasts and cook for 5-6 minutes on each side, or until golden brown and cooked through.
4. Pour the orange glaze over the chicken, reduce the heat, and simmer for 2-3 minutes until the sauce thickens.
5. Serve warm, drizzled with extra glaze.

Nutrition Info per Serving:
- Calories: 250
- Protein: 30g
- Carbohydrates: 10g
- Dietary Fiber: 0g
- Sugars: 8g
- Fat: 10g
- Saturated Fat: 2g
- Sodium: 150mg

Servings: 4
Cooking Time: 20 minutes

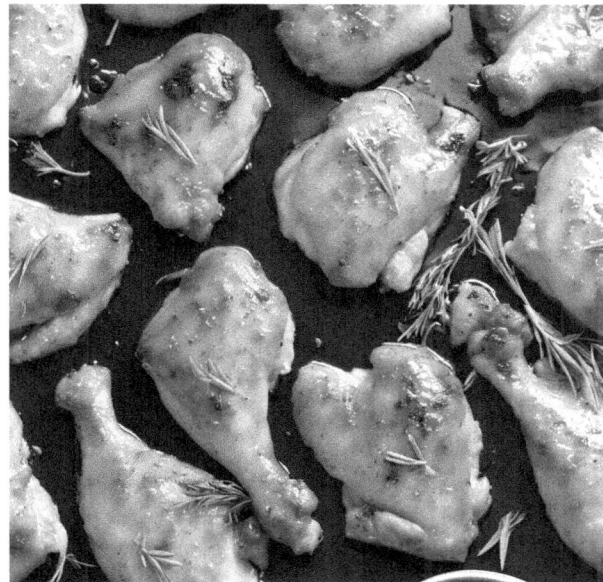

13. Turkey Lettuce Cups

Ingredients:
- 1 lb ground turkey (lean)
- 1 tbsp olive oil
- 1 onion, finely chopped
- 2 cloves garlic, minced
- 1 red bell pepper, finely chopped
- 2 tbsp low-sodium soy sauce
- 1 tbsp hoisin sauce (optional, if tolerated)
- 1/2 tsp ground black pepper
- 1/4 cup water chestnuts, chopped
- 1 head butter lettuce, leaves separated
- 2 green onions, chopped

Instructions:
1. In a large skillet, heat the olive oil over medium heat.
2. Add the onion and cook until softened, about 3-4 minutes.
3. Add the garlic and cook for another minute.
4. Add the ground turkey and cook until browned, about 5-7 minutes.
5. Stir in the red bell pepper, soy sauce, hoisin sauce (if using), and black pepper. Cook for another 3-4 minutes.
6. Stir in the water chestnuts and cook for an additional 2 minutes.
7. Spoon the turkey mixture into lettuce leaves and top with chopped green onions.
8. Serve immediately.

Nutrition Info per Serving:
- Calories: 210
- Protein: 24g
- Carbohydrates: 8g
- Dietary Fiber: 2g
- Sugars: 4g
- Fat: 10g
- Saturated Fat: 2g
- Sodium: 200mg

Servings: 4
Cooking Time: 20 minutes

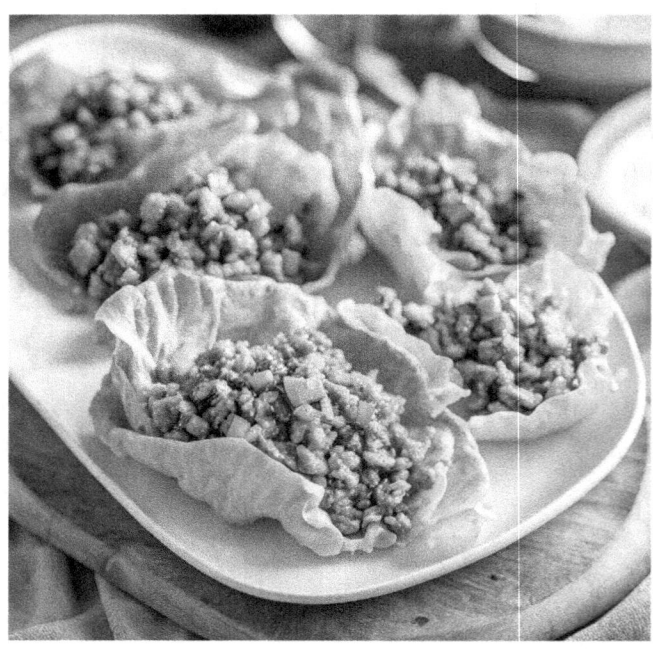

14. Chicken and Spinach Stew

Ingredients:
- 1 lb boneless, skinless chicken thighs, cut into bite-sized pieces
- 1 tbsp olive oil
- 1 onion, chopped
- 2 cloves garlic, minced
- 2 cups low-sodium chicken broth
- 1 can (14.5 oz) diced tomatoes, no salt added
- 1 tsp dried basil
- 1/2 tsp ground black pepper
- 4 cups fresh spinach, chopped

Instructions:
1. In a large pot, heat the olive oil over medium heat.
2. Add the onion and cook until softened, about 3-4 minutes.
3. Add the garlic and cook for another minute.
4. Add the chicken and cook until browned, about 5-7 minutes.
5. Stir in the chicken broth, diced tomatoes, basil, and black pepper. Bring to a boil.
6. Reduce heat and simmer for 20 minutes.
7. Stir in the chopped spinach and cook until wilted, about 2 minutes.
8. Serve warm.

Nutrition Info per Serving:
- Calories: 180
- Protein: 24g
- Carbohydrates: 8g
- Dietary Fiber: 2g
- Sugars: 4g
- Fat: 6g
- Saturated Fat: 1.5g
- Sodium: 180mg

Servings: 4
Cooking Time: 30 minutes

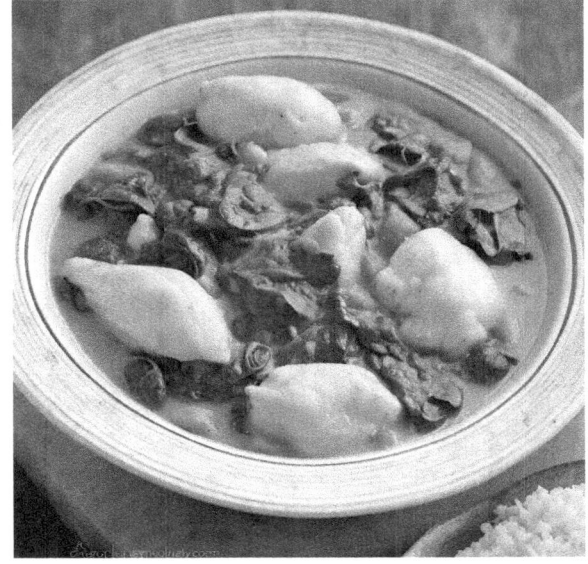

15. Turkey Quinoa Stuffed Peppers

Ingredients:
- 4 bell peppers, tops cut off and seeds removed
- 1 lb ground turkey (lean)
- 1 tbsp olive oil
- 1 onion, chopped
- 2 cloves garlic, minced
- 1 cup cooked quinoa
- 1 can (14.5 oz) diced tomatoes, no salt added
- 1 tsp dried oregano
- 1/2 tsp ground black pepper
- 1/4 cup fresh parsley, chopped

Instructions:
1. Preheat the oven to 375°F (190°C).
2. In a large skillet, heat the olive oil over medium heat.
3. Add the onion and cook until softened, about 3-4 minutes.
4. Add the garlic and cook for another minute.
5. Add the ground turkey and cook until browned, about 5-7 minutes.
6. Stir in the cooked quinoa, diced tomatoes, oregano, and black pepper. Cook for another 3-4 minutes.
7. Remove from heat and stir in the fresh parsley.
8. Stuff each bell pepper with the turkey and quinoa mixture.
9. Place the stuffed peppers in a baking dish and bake in the preheated oven for 25-30 minutes, or until the peppers are tender.
10. Serve warm.

Nutrition Info per Serving:
- Calories: 250
- Protein: 22g
- Carbohydrates: 25g
- Dietary Fiber: 5g
- Sugars: 8g
- Fat: 8g
- Saturated Fat: 1.5g
- Sodium: 180mg

Servings: 4
Cooking Time: 40 minutes

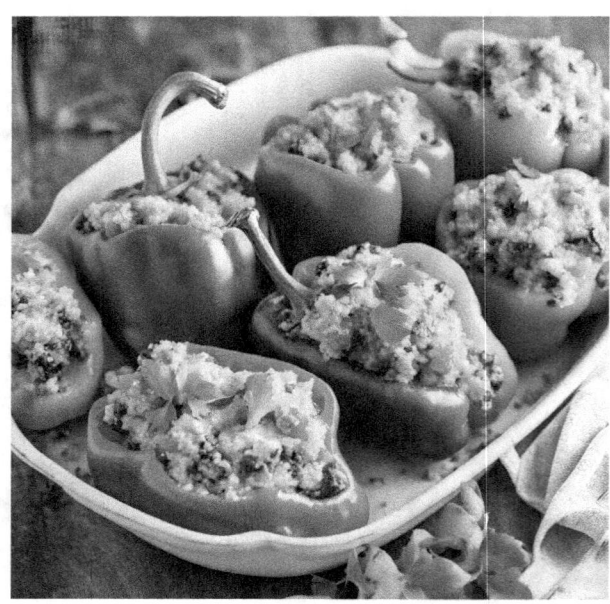

16. Chicken Cauliflower Fried Rice

Ingredients:
- 1 lb boneless, skinless chicken breast, diced
- 1 medium head cauliflower, grated (to resemble rice)
- 2 tbsp olive oil
- 1 onion, chopped
- 2 cloves garlic, minced
- 1 cup frozen peas and carrots
- 2 eggs, lightly beaten
- 3 tbsp low-sodium soy sauce
- 1/2 tsp ground black pepper
- 2 green onions, chopped

Instructions:
1. Heat 1 tbsp olive oil in a large skillet over medium heat. Add the chicken and cook until browned and cooked through, about 5-7 minutes. Remove from the skillet and set aside.
2. Add the remaining 1 tbsp olive oil to the skillet. Add the onion and garlic, and cook until softened, about 3-4 minutes.
3. Stir in the grated cauliflower and frozen peas and carrots. Cook for another 5 minutes until the vegetables are tender.
4. Push the vegetables to one side of the skillet. Pour the beaten eggs into the empty side and scramble until fully cooked.
5. Stir everything together and add the cooked chicken back to the skillet.
6. Add the soy sauce and ground black pepper, stirring to combine.
7. Cook for another 2-3 minutes until heated through.
8. Garnish with chopped green onions and serve warm.

Nutrition Info per Serving:
- Calories: 250
- Protein: 28g
- Carbohydrates: 12g
- Dietary Fiber: 4g
- Sugars: 4g
- Fat: 10g
- Saturated Fat: 2g
- Sodium: 320mg

Servings: 4
Cooking Time: 25 minutes

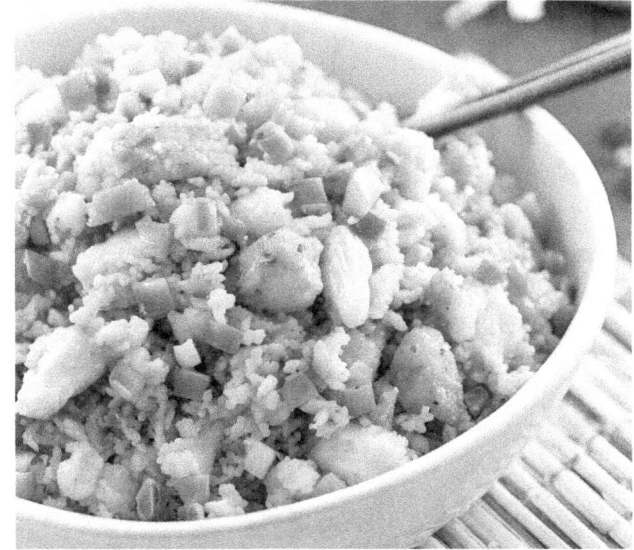

17. Chicken Broth with Parsley

Ingredients:
- 1 whole chicken (3-4 lbs), giblets removed
- 10 cups water
- 2 onions, quartered
- 3 carrots, chopped
- 3 celery stalks, chopped
- 4 cloves garlic, peeled and smashed
- 1 bay leaf
- 1/2 tsp ground black pepper
- 1/4 cup fresh parsley, chopped

Instructions:
1. Place the chicken in a large pot. Add the water, onions, carrots, celery, garlic, bay leaf, and ground black pepper.
2. Bring to a boil over high heat, then reduce the heat to low and simmer for 2-3 hours, skimming any foam that rises to the surface.
3. Remove the chicken from the pot. Let it cool slightly, then remove the meat from the bones and shred it. Set aside.
4. Strain the broth through a fine-mesh sieve into another large pot, discarding the solids.
5. Stir in the chopped parsley.
6. Serve warm, with the shredded chicken added back into the broth if desired.

Nutrition Info per Serving:
- Calories: 150
- Protein: 18g
- Carbohydrates: 6g
- Dietary Fiber: 2g
- Sugars: 3g
- Fat: 5g
- Saturated Fat: 1.5g
- Sodium: 100mg

Servings: 8
Cooking Time: 3 hours

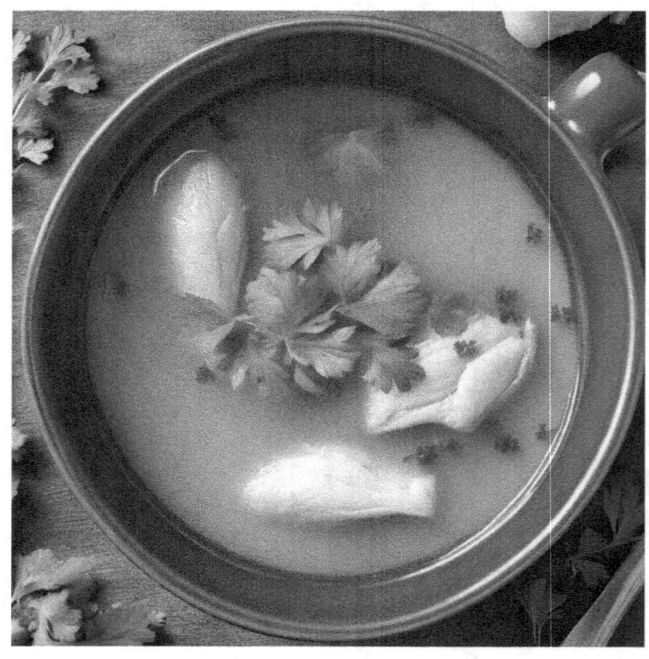

18. Turkey and Sweet Potato Skillet

Ingredients:
- 1 lb ground turkey (lean)
- 1 tbsp olive oil
- 1 onion, chopped
- 2 cloves garlic, minced
- 2 medium sweet potatoes, peeled and diced
- 1 red bell pepper, chopped
- 1 tsp ground cumin
- 1/2 tsp ground black pepper
- 1/4 tsp ground cinnamon
- 1/4 cup fresh cilantro, chopped

Instructions:
1. Heat the olive oil in a large skillet over medium heat. Add the onion and garlic, and cook until softened, about 3-4 minutes.
2. Add the ground turkey and cook until browned, about 5-7 minutes.
3. Stir in the sweet potatoes, red bell pepper, cumin, black pepper, and cinnamon. Cook for another 10-12 minutes until the sweet potatoes are tender.
4. Sprinkle with fresh cilantro and serve warm.

Nutrition Info per Serving:
- Calories: 280
- Protein: 24g
- Carbohydrates: 28g
- Dietary Fiber: 6g
- Sugars: 8g
- Fat: 10g
- Saturated Fat: 2g
- Sodium: 150mg

Servings: 4
Cooking Time: 25 minutes

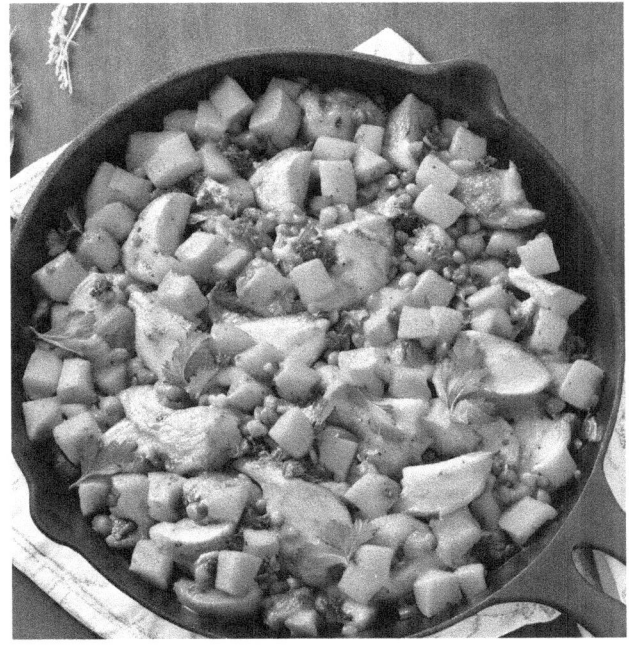

19. Chicken Piccata

Ingredients:
- 4 boneless, skinless chicken breasts
- 1/4 cup whole wheat flour
- 2 tbsp olive oil
- 1/4 cup lemon juice
- 1/2 cup low-sodium chicken broth
- 2 tbsp capers, rinsed and drained
- 1/2 tsp ground black pepper
- 1 tbsp fresh parsley, chopped

Instructions:
1. Lightly coat the chicken breasts with the whole wheat flour, shaking off any excess.
2. Heat the olive oil in a large skillet over medium-high heat. Add the chicken breasts and cook until golden brown, about 4-5 minutes per side. Remove from the skillet and set aside.
3. In the same skillet, add the lemon juice, chicken broth, capers, and ground black pepper. Bring to a boil, scraping up any browned bits from the bottom of the skillet.
4. Return the chicken to the skillet and simmer for another 5 minutes, until the sauce has thickened slightly and the chicken is cooked through.
5. Sprinkle with fresh parsley and serve warm.

Nutrition Info per Serving:
- Calories: 220
- Protein: 28g
- Carbohydrates: 8g
- Dietary Fiber: 2g
- Sugars: 1g
- Fat: 9g
- Saturated Fat: 1.5g
- Sodium: 200mg

Servings: 4
Cooking Time: 20 minutes

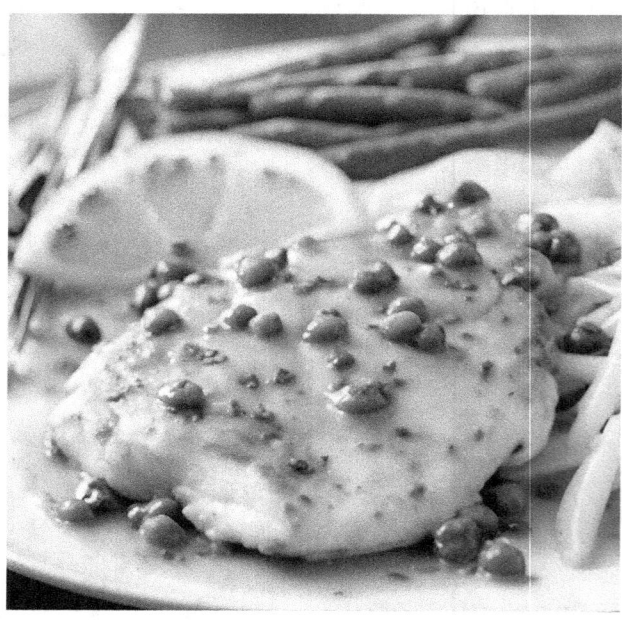

20. Chicken Ratatouille

Ingredients:
- 1 lb boneless, skinless chicken thighs, cut into bite-sized pieces
- 2 tbsp olive oil
- 1 onion, chopped
- 2 cloves garlic, minced
- 1 eggplant, diced
- 1 zucchini, diced
- 1 red bell pepper, chopped
- 1 can (14.5 oz) diced tomatoes, no salt added
- 1 tsp dried basil
- 1/2 tsp ground black pepper
- 1/4 cup fresh basil, chopped

Instructions:
1. Heat 1 tbsp olive oil in a large pot over medium heat. Add the chicken thighs and cook until browned, about 5-7 minutes. Remove from the pot and set aside.
2. Add the remaining 1 tbsp olive oil to the pot. Add the onion and garlic, and cook until softened, about 3-4 minutes.
3. Stir in the eggplant, zucchini, and red bell pepper. Cook for another 5 minutes.
4. Add the diced tomatoes, dried basil, and black pepper. Bring to a boil.
5. Reduce heat and simmer for 20 minutes.
6. Return the chicken to the pot and simmer for another 5 minutes.
7. Stir in the fresh basil and serve warm.

Nutrition Info per Serving:
- Calories: 230
- Protein: 22g
- Carbohydrates: 15g
- Dietary Fiber: 5g
- Sugars: 9g
- Fat: 10g
- Saturated Fat: 2g
- Sodium: 200mg

Servings: 4
Cooking Time: 35 minutes

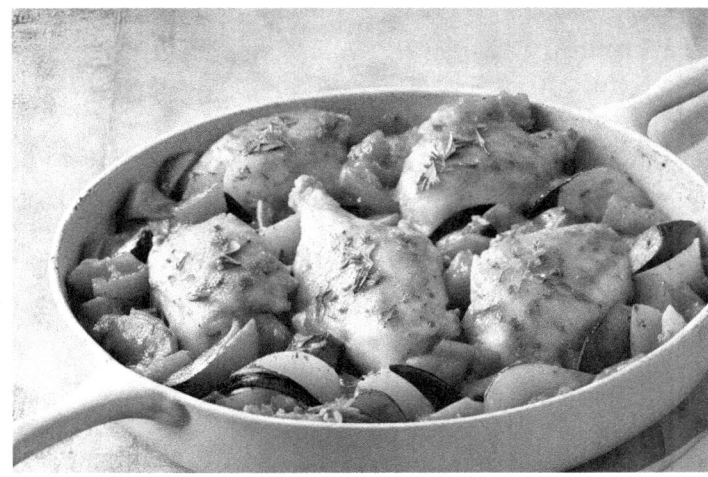

21. Grilled Chicken with Peach Salsa

Ingredients:
- 4 boneless, skinless chicken breasts
- 1 tbsp olive oil
- 1/2 tsp ground black pepper
- 2 peaches, diced
- 1/4 red onion, finely chopped
- 1 jalapeño, seeded and finely chopped (optional)
- 1 tbsp fresh cilantro, chopped
- 1 tbsp lime juice

Instructions:
1. Preheat the grill to medium-high heat.
2. Brush the chicken breasts with olive oil and sprinkle with ground black pepper.
3. Grill the chicken for 6-7 minutes on each side, or until cooked through and the internal temperature reaches 165°F (74°C).
4. While the chicken is grilling, prepare the peach salsa by combining the diced peaches, red onion, jalapeño (if using), cilantro, and lime juice in a bowl. Mix well.
5. Serve the grilled chicken topped with peach salsa.

Nutrition Info per Serving:
- Calories: 210
- Protein: 28g
- Carbohydrates: 10g
- Dietary Fiber: 2g
- Sugars: 8g
- Fat: 7g
- Saturated Fat: 1.5g
- Sodium: 100mg

Servings: 4
Cooking Time: 15 minutes

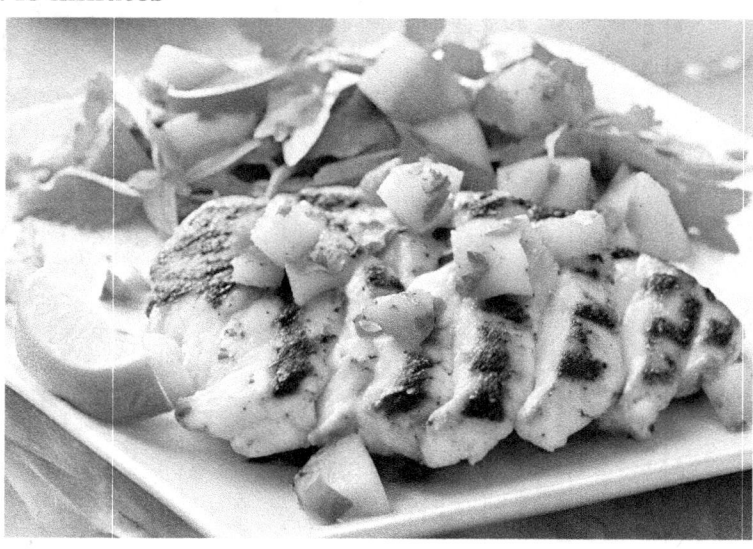

22. Chicken and Asparagus Lemon Stir Fry

Ingredients:
- 1 lb boneless, skinless chicken breast, sliced into thin strips
- 1 bunch asparagus, trimmed and cut into 2-inch pieces
- 1 tbsp olive oil
- 2 cloves garlic, minced
- 1/2 tsp ground black pepper
- 1 lemon, juiced and zested
- 1 tbsp low-sodium soy sauce
- 1 tbsp fresh parsley, chopped

Instructions:
1. Heat the olive oil in a large skillet or wok over medium-high heat.
2. Add the chicken strips and cook until browned and cooked through, about 5-7 minutes.
3. Add the garlic and asparagus, and stir-fry for another 3-4 minutes until the asparagus is tender-crisp.
4. Stir in the lemon juice, lemon zest, soy sauce, and ground black pepper. Cook for another 1-2 minutes until heated through.
5. Garnish with fresh parsley and serve warm.

Nutrition Info per Serving:
- Calories: 220
- Protein: 28g
- Carbohydrates: 8g
- Dietary Fiber: 3g
- Sugars: 3g
- Fat: 9g
- Saturated Fat: 1.5g
- Sodium: 180mg

Servings: 4
Cooking Time: 15 minutes

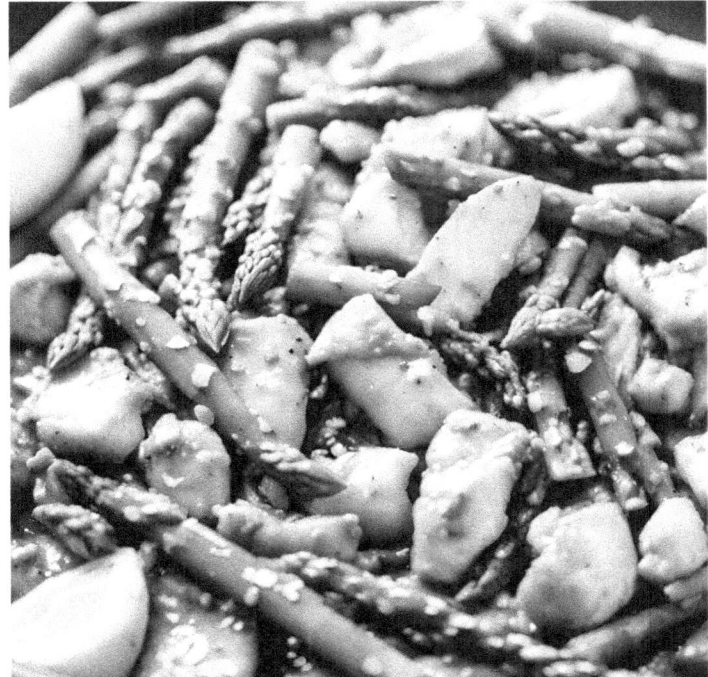

23. Minty Turkey Patties

Ingredients:
- 1 lb ground turkey (lean)
- 1/4 cup whole wheat breadcrumbs
- 1 large egg white
- 2 tbsp fresh mint, chopped
- 2 cloves garlic, minced
- 1/2 tsp ground black pepper
- 1 tbsp olive oil (for cooking)

Instructions:
1. In a large bowl, mix together the ground turkey, breadcrumbs, egg white, mint, garlic, and ground black pepper until well combined.
2. Shape the mixture into 8 small patties.
3. Heat the olive oil in a large skillet over medium heat.
4. Cook the patties for 4-5 minutes per side, or until cooked through and golden brown.
5. Serve warm.

Nutrition Info per Serving:
- Calories: 180
- Protein: 22g
- Carbohydrates: 5g
- Dietary Fiber: 1g
- Sugars: 0g
- Fat: 8g
- Saturated Fat: 2g
- Sodium: 120mg

Servings: 4
Cooking Time: 15 minutes

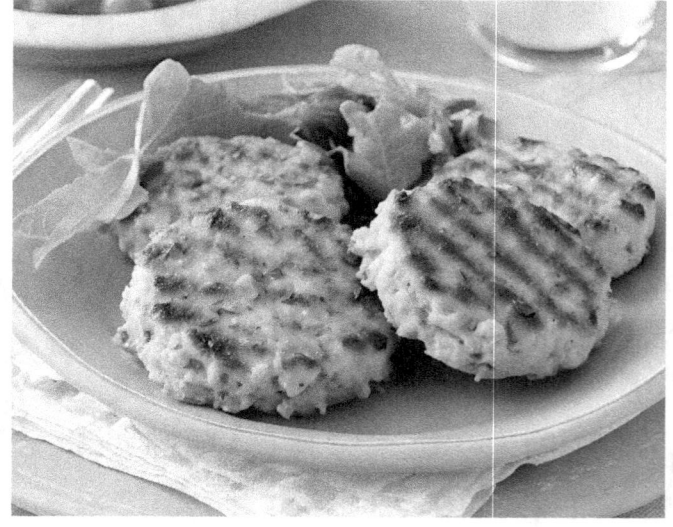

24. Chicken Pepperoni Marinara

Ingredients:
- 4 boneless, skinless chicken breasts
- 1 tbsp olive oil
- 1/2 cup turkey pepperoni slices, cut into halves
- 1 onion, chopped
- 2 cloves garlic, minced
- 1 can (14.5 oz) diced tomatoes, no salt added
- 1/2 cup low-sodium marinara sauce
- 1 tsp dried basil
- 1/2 tsp ground black pepper
- 1/4 cup fresh basil, chopped

Instructions:
1. Preheat the oven to 375°F (190°C).
2. Heat the olive oil in a large oven-safe skillet over medium heat.
3. Add the chicken breasts and cook until golden brown, about 4-5 minutes per side. Remove from the skillet and set aside.
4. In the same skillet, add the turkey pepperoni, onion, and garlic. Cook for 3-4 minutes until the onion is softened.
5. Stir in the diced tomatoes, marinara sauce, dried basil, and ground black pepper. Bring to a simmer.
6. Return the chicken to the skillet and spoon some of the sauce over the top.
7. Transfer the skillet to the preheated oven and bake for 20 minutes, or until the chicken is cooked through.
8. Garnish with fresh basil and serve warm.

Nutrition Info per Serving:
- Calories: 250
- Protein: 30g
- Carbohydrates: 10g
- Dietary Fiber: 3g
- Sugars: 5g
- Fat: 10g
- Saturated Fat: 2g
- Sodium: 200mg

Servings: 4
Cooking Time: 30 minutes

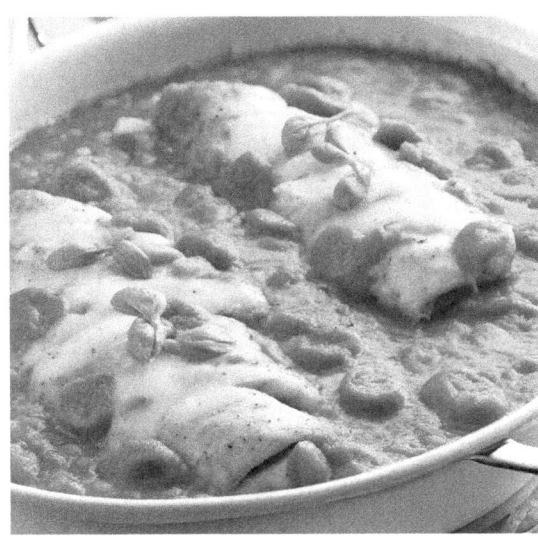

25. Sage Turkey Loaf

Ingredients:
- 1 lb ground turkey (lean)
- 1/2 cup whole wheat breadcrumbs
- 1 large egg white
- 1 onion, finely chopped
- 2 cloves garlic, minced
- 1 tbsp fresh sage, chopped
- 1/2 tsp ground black pepper
- 1 tbsp olive oil (for brushing)

Instructions:
1. Preheat the oven to 350°F (175°C). Lightly grease a loaf pan.
2. In a large bowl, mix together the ground turkey, breadcrumbs, egg white, onion, garlic, sage, and ground black pepper until well combined.
3. Press the mixture into the prepared loaf pan and brush the top with olive oil.
4. Bake in the preheated oven for 45-50 minutes, or until the internal temperature reaches 165°F (74°C).
5. Let the turkey loaf rest for 10 minutes before slicing.
6. Serve warm.

Nutrition Info per Serving:
- Calories: 220
- Protein: 24g
- Carbohydrates: 10g
- Dietary Fiber: 2g
- Sugars: 3g
- Fat: 10g
- Saturated Fat: 2g
- Sodium: 150mg

Servings: 4
Cooking Time: 50 minutes

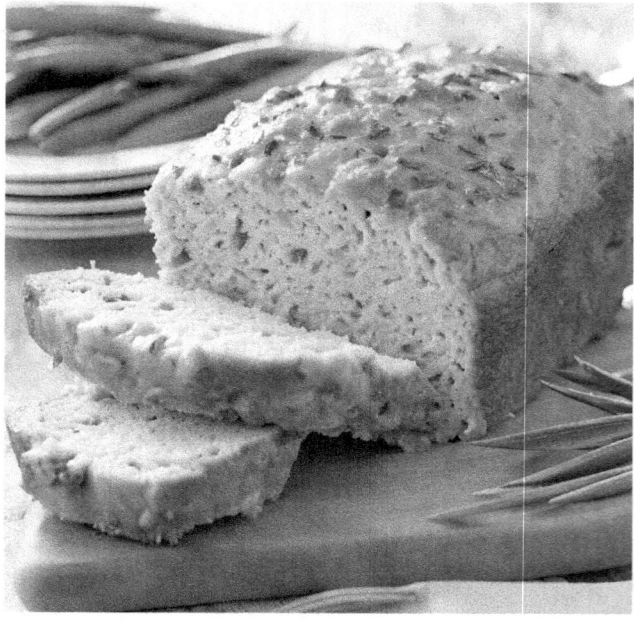

26. Chicken and Mushroom Casserole

Ingredients:
- 1 lb boneless, skinless chicken thighs, cut into bite-sized pieces
- 1 tbsp olive oil
- 1 onion, chopped
- 2 cloves garlic, minced
- 2 cups mushrooms, sliced
- 1 cup low-sodium chicken broth
- 1/2 cup skim milk
- 1/2 tsp ground black pepper
- 1/2 tsp dried thyme
- 1/4 cup whole wheat flour

Instructions:
1. Preheat the oven to 375°F (190°C).
2. Heat the olive oil in a large skillet over medium heat. Add the chicken thighs and cook until browned, about 5-7 minutes. Remove from the skillet and set aside.
3. In the same skillet, add the onion, garlic, and mushrooms. Cook until softened, about 3-4 minutes.
4. Sprinkle the whole wheat flour over the vegetables and stir to coat.
5. Gradually add the chicken broth and skim milk, stirring constantly until the mixture thickens.
6. Stir in the ground black pepper and dried thyme.
7. Return the chicken to the skillet and stir to combine.
8. Transfer the mixture to a baking dish and bake in the preheated oven for 25-30 minutes, or until bubbly and heated through.
9. Serve warm.

Nutrition Info per Serving:
- Calories: 250
- Protein: 28g
- Carbohydrates: 15g
- Dietary Fiber: 3g
- Sugars: 5g
- Fat: 9g
- Saturated Fat: 2g
- Sodium: 180mg

Servings: 4
Cooking Time: 35 minutes

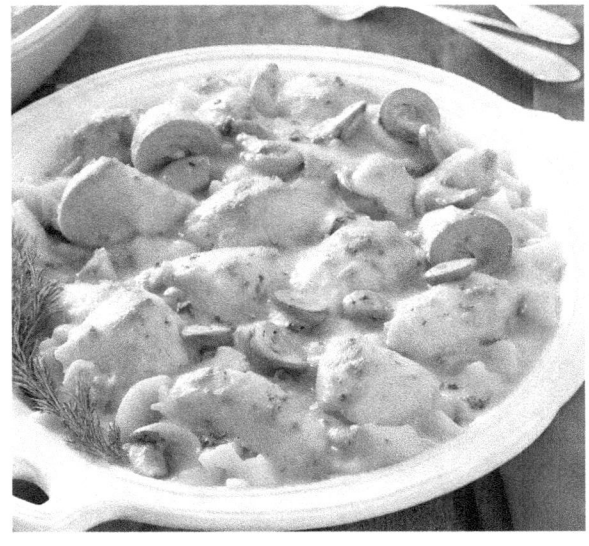

27. Grilled Turkey and Pineapple

Ingredients:
- 4 turkey breast cutlets
- 1 tbsp olive oil
- 1/2 tsp ground black pepper
- 1 pineapple, peeled, cored, and sliced into rings
- 1 tbsp fresh cilantro, chopped

Instructions:
1. Preheat the grill to medium-high heat.
2. Brush the turkey cutlets with olive oil and sprinkle with ground black pepper.
3. Grill the turkey cutlets for 4-5 minutes per side, or until cooked through and the internal temperature reaches 165°F (74°C).
4. While the turkey is grilling, place the pineapple rings on the grill and cook for 2-3 minutes per side until lightly charred.
5. Serve the grilled turkey with pineapple rings, garnished with fresh cilantro.

Nutrition Info per Serving:
- Calories: 220
- Protein: 28g
- Carbohydrates: 12g
- Dietary Fiber: 2g
- Sugars: 10g
- Fat: 7g
- Saturated Fat: 1.5g
- Sodium: 100mg

Servings: 4
Cooking Time: 15 minutes

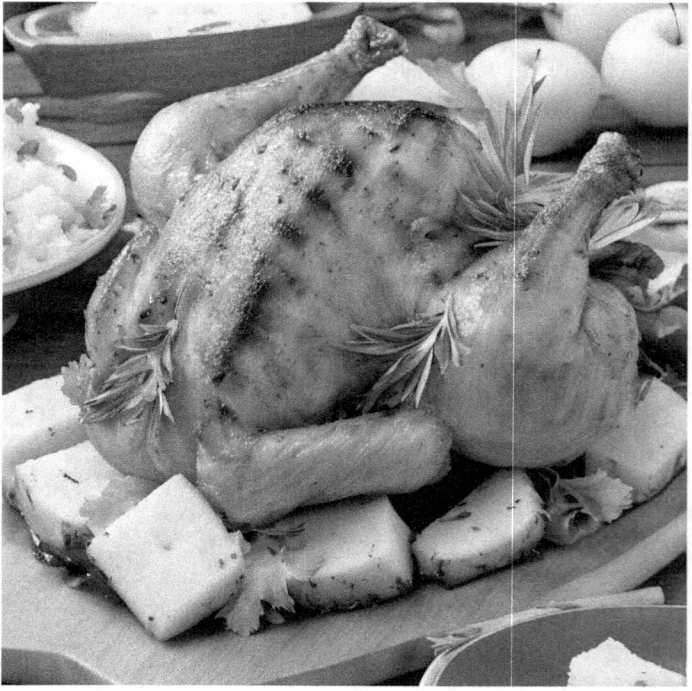

28. Chicken and Broccoli Alfredo

Ingredients:
- 1 lb boneless, skinless chicken breast, sliced into strips
- 1 tbsp olive oil
- 2 cloves garlic, minced
- 2 cups broccoli florets
- 1 cup skim milk
- 1/2 cup low-fat Parmesan cheese, grated
- 1 tbsp whole wheat flour
- 1/2 tsp ground black pepper
- 1/2 tsp dried basil
- 8 oz whole wheat fettuccine, cooked according to package instructions

Instructions:
1. Heat the olive oil in a large skillet over medium heat. Add the chicken strips and cook until browned and cooked through, about 5-7 minutes. Remove from the skillet and set aside.
2. In the same skillet, add the garlic and broccoli. Cook until the broccoli is tender, about 3-4 minutes.
3. Sprinkle the whole wheat flour over the broccoli and stir to coat.
4. Gradually add the skim milk, stirring constantly until the mixture thickens.
5. Stir in the grated Parmesan cheese, ground black pepper, and dried basil.
6. Return the chicken to the skillet and stir to combine.
7. Toss the cooked fettuccine with the Alfredo sauce.
8. Serve warm.

Nutrition Info per Serving:
- Calories: 350
- Protein: 30g
- Carbohydrates: 40g
- Dietary Fiber: 6g
- Sugars: 5g
- Fat: 10g
- Saturated Fat: 3g
- Sodium: 250mg

Servings: 4
Cooking Time: 20 minutes

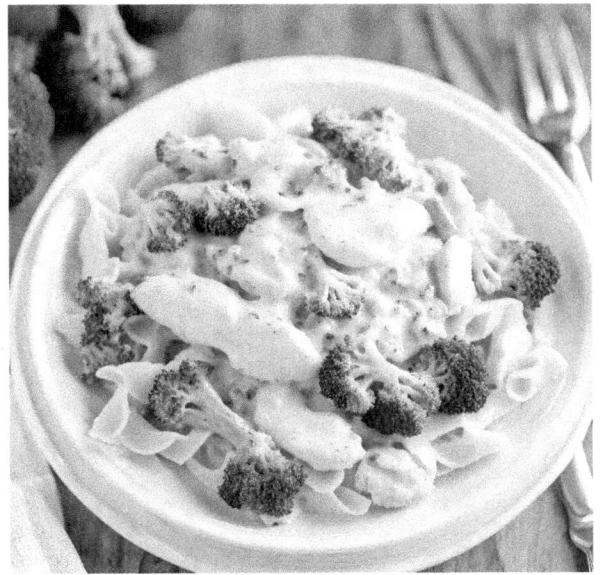

29. Chicken Fajitas

Ingredients:
- 1 lb boneless, skinless chicken breast, sliced into strips
- 2 tbsp olive oil
- 1 red bell pepper, sliced
- 1 yellow bell pepper, sliced
- 1 onion, sliced
- 2 cloves garlic, minced
- 1 tsp ground cumin
- 1/2 tsp ground black pepper
- 1/2 tsp ground paprika
- 8 whole wheat tortillas
- 1/4 cup fresh cilantro, chopped
- 1 lime, cut into wedges

Instructions:
1. Heat 1 tbsp olive oil in a large skillet over medium heat. Add the chicken strips and cook until browned and cooked through, about 5-7 minutes. Remove from the skillet and set aside.
2. Add the remaining 1 tbsp olive oil to the skillet. Add the bell peppers, onion, and garlic. Cook until the vegetables are tender, about 5-7 minutes.
3. Stir in the ground cumin, black pepper, and paprika.
4. Return the chicken to the skillet and stir to combine. Cook for another 2-3 minutes until heated through.
5. Serve the chicken and vegetables in whole wheat tortillas, garnished with fresh cilantro and lime wedges.

Nutrition Info per Serving:
- Calories: 300
- Protein: 26g
- Carbohydrates: 30g
- Dietary Fiber: 5g
- Sugars: 4g
- Fat: 10g
- Saturated Fat: 2g
- Sodium: 200mg

Servings: 4
Cooking Time: 20 minutes

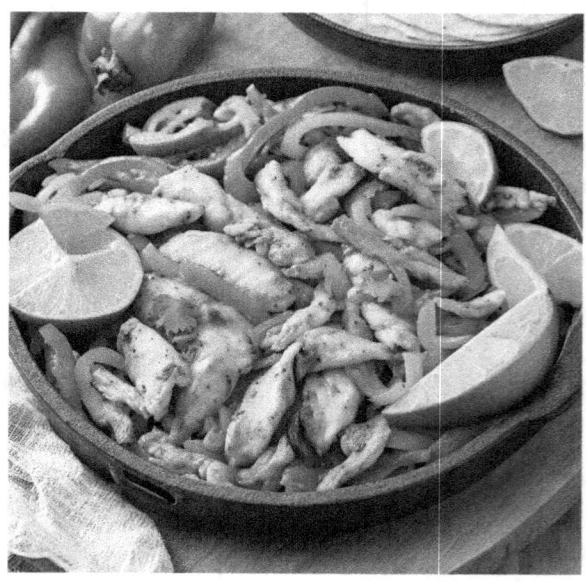

30. Turkey and Parsnip Mash

Ingredients:
- 1 lb ground turkey (lean)
- 1 tbsp olive oil
- 1 onion, chopped
- 2 cloves garlic, minced
- 4 parsnips, peeled and chopped
- 2 cups low-sodium chicken broth
- 1/2 tsp ground black pepper
- 1/4 cup fresh parsley, chopped

Instructions:
1. In a large pot, bring the parsnips and chicken broth to a boil. Reduce heat and simmer until the parsnips are tender, about 15-20 minutes.
2. While the parsnips are cooking, heat the olive oil in a large skillet over medium heat. Add the onion and garlic, and cook until softened, about 3-4 minutes.
3. Add the ground turkey and cook until browned, about 5-7 minutes. Stir in the ground black pepper.
4. Drain the parsnips, reserving 1/2 cup of the cooking liquid.
5. Mash the parsnips, adding the reserved cooking liquid as needed to achieve a smooth consistency.
6. Stir in the fresh parsley.
7. Serve the ground turkey over the parsnip mash.

Nutrition Info per Serving:
- Calories: 250
- Protein: 25g
- Carbohydrates: 25g
- Dietary Fiber: 6g
- Sugars: 6g
- Fat: 8g
- Saturated Fat: 2g
- Sodium: 200mg

Servings: 4
Cooking Time: 25 minutes

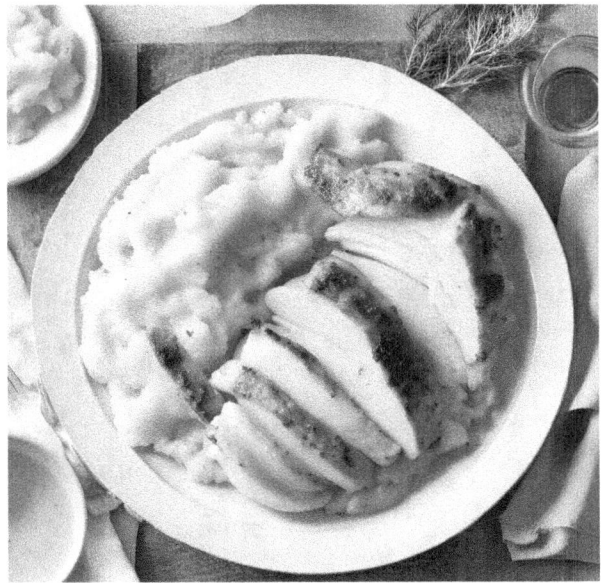

Fish and Seafood Recipes

1. Grilled Salmon with Dill
Ingredients:
- 4 salmon fillets (about 6 oz each)
- 2 tbsp olive oil
- 1 lemon, juiced and zested
- 2 tbsp fresh dill, chopped
- 2 cloves garlic, minced
- 1/2 tsp ground black pepper

Instructions:
1. Preheat the grill to medium-high heat.
2. In a small bowl, mix together the olive oil, lemon juice, lemon zest, dill, garlic, and ground black pepper.
3. Brush the salmon fillets with the dill mixture.
4. Grill the salmon fillets for 4-5 minutes per side, or until the fish flakes easily with a fork.
5. Serve warm.

Nutrition Info per Serving:
- Calories: 300
- Protein: 34g
- Carbohydrates: 2g
- Dietary Fiber: 0g
- Sugars: 0g
- Fat: 18g
- Saturated Fat: 3g
- Sodium: 75mg

Servings: 4
Cooking Time: 10 minutes

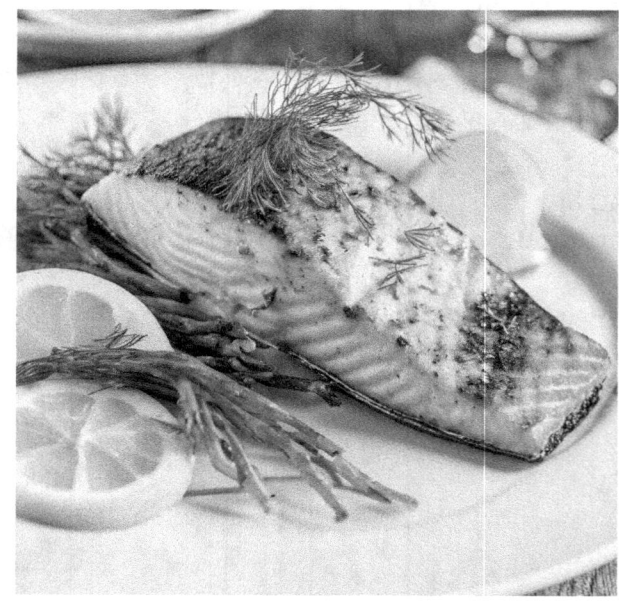

2. Poached Cod

Ingredients:
- 4 cod fillets (about 6 oz each)
- 4 cups low-sodium chicken broth
- 1 lemon, sliced
- 1 bay leaf
- 1/2 tsp ground black pepper
- 2 tbsp fresh parsley, chopped

Instructions:
1. In a large skillet, bring the chicken broth to a simmer.
2. Add the lemon slices, bay leaf, and ground black pepper.
3. Carefully place the cod fillets in the skillet.
4. Poach the cod for 6-8 minutes, or until the fish is opaque and flakes easily with a fork.
5. Remove the cod from the skillet and discard the bay leaf.
6. Serve the poached cod garnished with fresh parsley.

Nutrition Info per Serving:
- Calories: 150
- Protein: 32g
- Carbohydrates: 2g
- Dietary Fiber: 0g
- Sugars: 0g
- Fat: 1g
- Saturated Fat: 0g
- Sodium: 220mg

Servings: 4
Cooking Time: 10 minutes

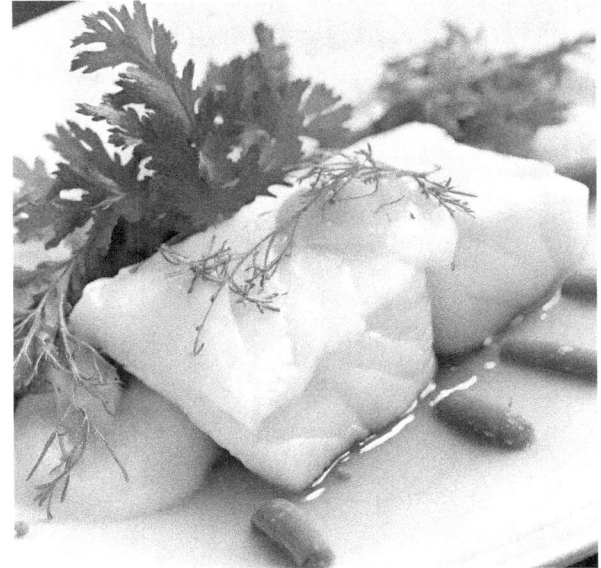

3. Baked Tilapia with Lemon Pepper

Ingredients:
- 4 tilapia fillets (about 6 oz each)
- 2 tbsp olive oil
- 1 lemon, juiced and zested
- 1 tsp ground black pepper
- 1 tsp dried oregano
- 1/2 tsp garlic powder
- 1 tbsp fresh parsley, chopped

Instructions:
1. Preheat the oven to 375°F (190°C).
2. In a small bowl, mix together the olive oil, lemon juice, lemon zest, black pepper, oregano, and garlic powder.
3. Place the tilapia fillets in a baking dish and brush with the lemon pepper mixture.
4. Bake in the preheated oven for 15-20 minutes, or until the fish flakes easily with a fork.
5. Serve garnished with fresh parsley.

Nutrition Info per Serving:
- Calories: 220
- Protein: 35g
- Carbohydrates: 1g
- Dietary Fiber: 0g
- Sugars: 0g
- Fat: 8g
- Saturated Fat: 1.5g
- Sodium: 100mg

Servings: 4
Cooking Time: 20 minutes

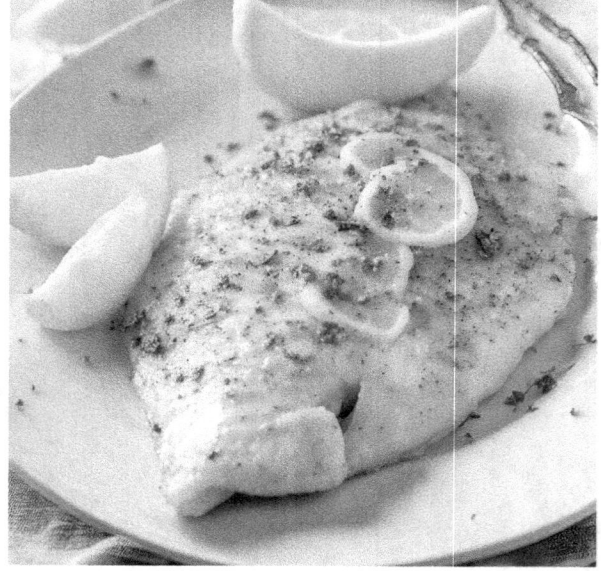

4. Shrimp and Vegetable Stir-Fry

Ingredients:
- 1 lb large shrimp, peeled and deveined
- 2 tbsp olive oil
- 1 red bell pepper, sliced
- 1 yellow bell pepper, sliced
- 1 zucchini, sliced
- 1 cup snow peas
- 2 cloves garlic, minced
- 1 tbsp low-sodium soy sauce
- 1/2 tsp ground ginger
- 1/2 tsp ground black pepper

Instructions:
1. Heat 1 tbsp olive oil in a large skillet or wok over medium-high heat.
2. Add the shrimp and cook until pink and opaque, about 2-3 minutes per side. Remove from the skillet and set aside.
3. Add the remaining 1 tbsp olive oil to the skillet. Add the bell peppers, zucchini, snow peas, and garlic. Stir-fry for 5-6 minutes until the vegetables are tender-crisp.
4. Stir in the soy sauce, ground ginger, and ground black pepper.
5. Return the shrimp to the skillet and stir-fry for another 2 minutes until heated through.
6. Serve warm.

Nutrition Info per Serving:
- Calories: 200
- Protein: 28g
- Carbohydrates: 8g
- Dietary Fiber: 3g
- Sugars: 4g
- Fat: 7g
- Saturated Fat: 1g
- Sodium: 300mg

Servings: 4
Cooking Time: 15 minutes

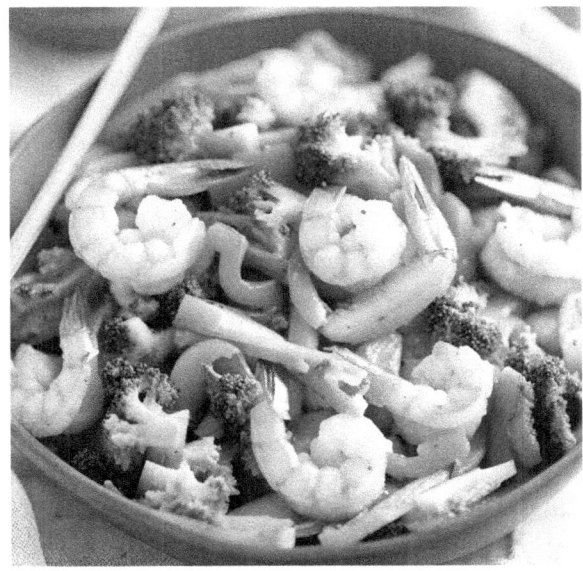

5. Steamed Mussels with Garlic and Herbs

Ingredients:
- 2 lbs mussels, cleaned and debearded
- 2 tbsp olive oil
- 4 cloves garlic, minced
- 1/2 cup low-sodium chicken broth
- 1/2 cup dry white wine (optional, can substitute with more broth)
- 1 tbsp lemon juice
- 1/2 tsp ground black pepper
- 2 tbsp fresh parsley, chopped
- 1 tbsp fresh thyme, chopped

Instructions:
1. Heat the olive oil in a large pot over medium heat. Add the garlic and cook until fragrant, about 1 minute.
2. Add the chicken broth, white wine (if using), lemon juice, and ground black pepper. Bring to a simmer.
3. Add the mussels to the pot, cover, and steam for 5-7 minutes, or until the mussels have opened. Discard any mussels that do not open.
4. Stir in the fresh parsley and thyme.
5. Serve the steamed mussels with the cooking liquid.

Nutrition Info per Serving:
- Calories: 250
- Protein: 32g
- Carbohydrates: 6g
- Dietary Fiber: 0g
- Sugars: 0g
- Fat: 10g
- Saturated Fat: 2g
- Sodium: 350mg

Servings: 4
Cooking Time: 10 minutes

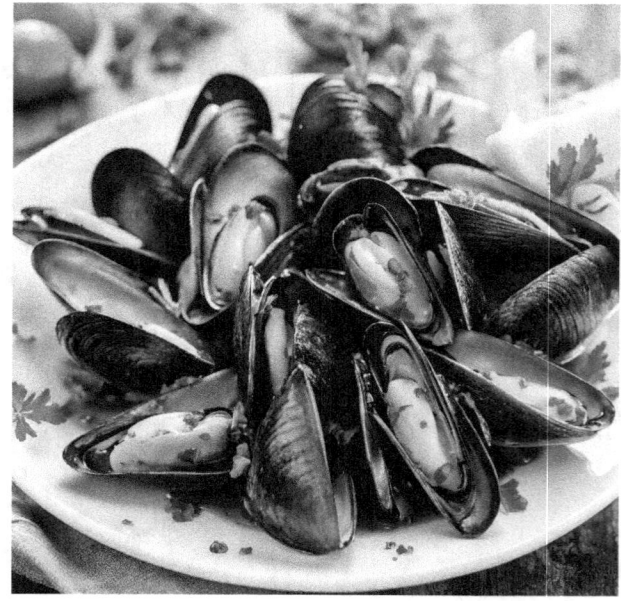

6. Crab Salad with Cucumber

Ingredients:
- 1 lb crab meat, cooked and shredded
- 1 cucumber, thinly sliced
- 1/4 cup red onion, finely chopped
- 2 tbsp olive oil
- 1 tbsp lemon juice
- 1 tsp Dijon mustard
- 1/2 tsp ground black pepper
- 2 tbsp fresh dill, chopped

Instructions:
1. In a large bowl, combine the crab meat, cucumber, and red onion.
2. In a small bowl, whisk together the olive oil, lemon juice, Dijon mustard, and ground black pepper.
3. Pour the dressing over the crab mixture and toss gently to combine.
4. Sprinkle with fresh dill and serve chilled.

Nutrition Info per Serving:
- Calories: 200
- Protein: 25g
- Carbohydrates: 5g
- Dietary Fiber: 1g
- Sugars: 2g
- Fat: 9g
- Saturated Fat: 1.5g
- Sodium: 320mg

Servings: 4
Cooking Time: 10 minutes

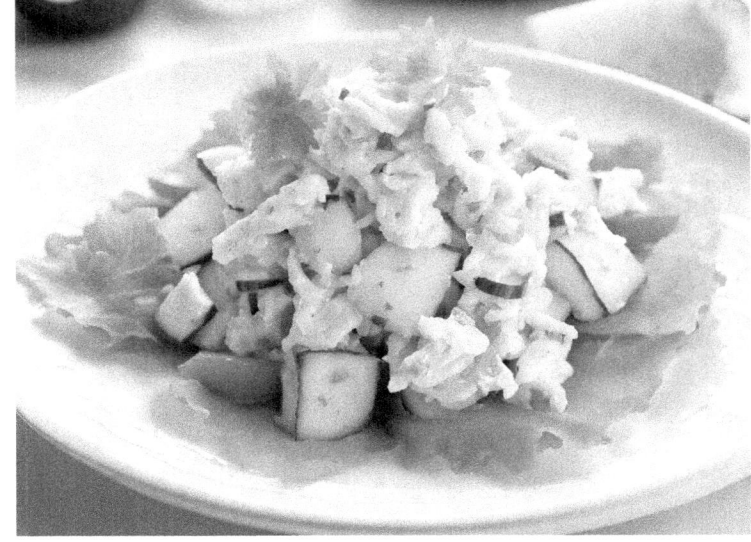

7. Fish Soup with Tomatoes

Ingredients:
- 1 lb white fish fillets (such as cod or haddock), cut into bite-sized pieces
- 1 tbsp olive oil
- 1 onion, chopped
- 2 cloves garlic, minced
- 4 cups low-sodium fish broth or chicken broth
- 1 can (14.5 oz) diced tomatoes, no salt added
- 1 tsp dried basil
- 1/2 tsp ground black pepper
- 1/4 cup fresh parsley, chopped

Instructions:
1. Heat the olive oil in a large pot over medium heat. Add the onion and garlic, and cook until softened, about 3-4 minutes.
2. Add the fish broth, diced tomatoes, dried basil, and ground black pepper. Bring to a boil.
3. Reduce heat and simmer for 10 minutes.
4. Add the fish pieces and cook for another 5-7 minutes, or until the fish is cooked through and opaque.
5. Stir in the fresh parsley and serve hot.

Nutrition Info per Serving:
- Calories: 180
- Protein: 25g
- Carbohydrates: 10g
- Dietary Fiber: 2g
- Sugars: 4g
- Fat: 5g
- Saturated Fat: 1g
- Sodium: 250mg

Servings: 4
Cooking Time: 25 minutes

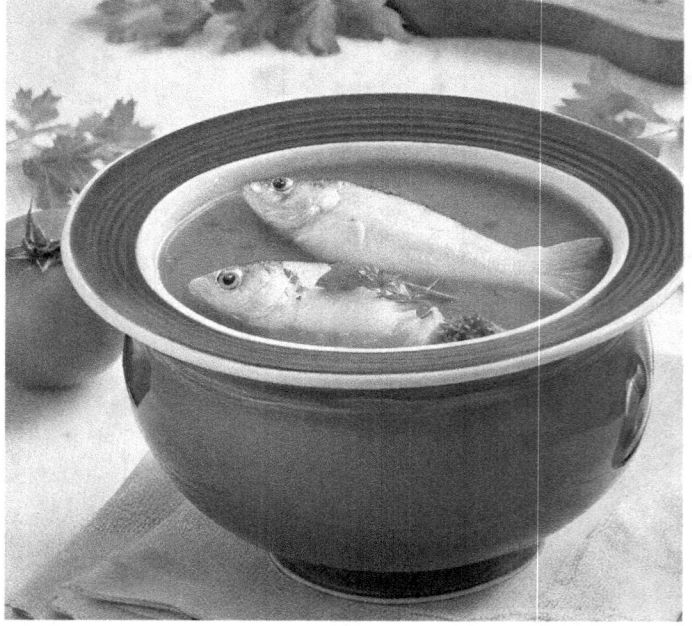

8. Baked Trout with Rosemary

Ingredients:
- 4 trout fillets (about 6 oz each)
- 2 tbsp olive oil
- 1 lemon, sliced
- 2 cloves garlic, minced
- 2 tbsp fresh rosemary, chopped
- 1/2 tsp ground black pepper

Instructions:
1. Preheat the oven to 375°F (190°C).
2. In a small bowl, mix together the olive oil, garlic, rosemary, and ground black pepper.
3. Place the trout fillets on a baking sheet lined with parchment paper. Brush the fillets with the olive oil mixture.
4. Arrange the lemon slices on top of the fillets.
5. Bake in the preheated oven for 15-20 minutes, or until the fish flakes easily with a fork.
6. Serve warm.

Nutrition Info per Serving:
- Calories: 250
- Protein: 34g
- Carbohydrates: 2g
- Dietary Fiber: 0g
- Sugars: 0g
- Fat: 11g
- Saturated Fat: 2g
- Sodium: 85mg

Servings: 4
Cooking Time: 20 minutes

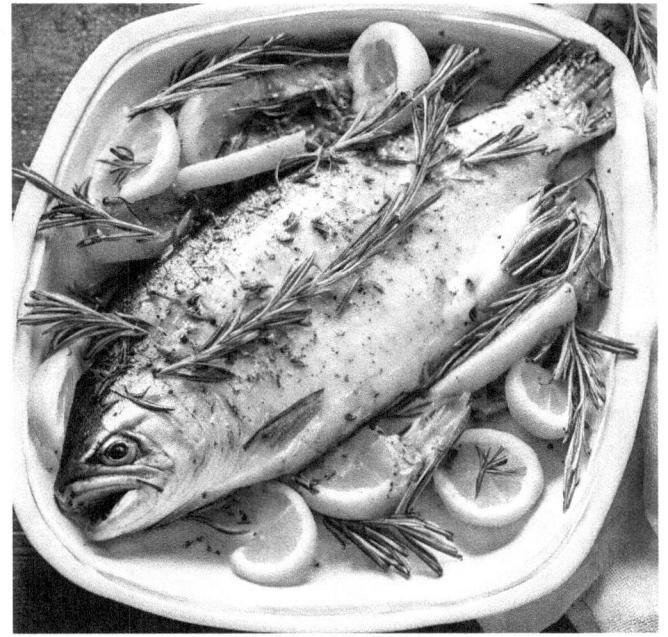

9. Grilled Shrimp Skewers

Ingredients:
- 1 lb large shrimp, peeled and deveined
- 2 tbsp olive oil
- 1 lemon, juiced
- 2 cloves garlic, minced
- 1 tsp paprika
- 1/2 tsp ground black pepper
- 2 tbsp fresh parsley, chopped

Instructions:
1. In a large bowl, combine the olive oil, lemon juice, garlic, paprika, and ground black pepper. Add the shrimp and toss to coat.
2. Thread the shrimp onto skewers.
3. Preheat the grill to medium-high heat.
4. Grill the shrimp skewers for 2-3 minutes per side, or until the shrimp are pink and opaque.
5. Garnish with fresh parsley and serve warm.

Nutrition Info per Serving:
- Calories: 180
- Protein: 28g
- Carbohydrates: 2g
- Dietary Fiber: 0g
- Sugars: 0g
- Fat: 6g
- Saturated Fat: 1g
- Sodium: 320mg

Servings: 4
Cooking Time: 10 minutes

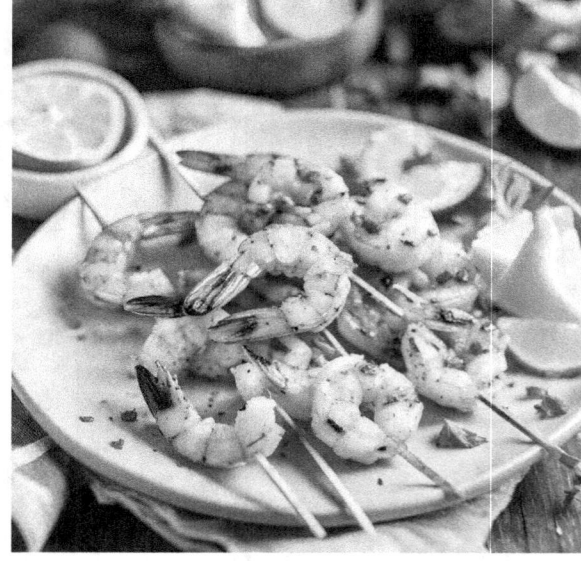

10. Scallops with Ginger and Soy

Ingredients:
- 1 lb sea scallops
- 2 tbsp olive oil
- 2 tbsp low-sodium soy sauce
- 1 tbsp fresh ginger, grated
- 2 cloves garlic, minced
- 1 tbsp lemon juice
- 1/2 tsp ground black pepper
- 2 green onions, chopped

Instructions:
1. Pat the scallops dry with a paper towel.
2. In a large skillet, heat the olive oil over medium-high heat.
3. Add the scallops and cook for 2-3 minutes per side, until they are golden brown and cooked through. Remove from the skillet and set aside.
4. In the same skillet, add the soy sauce, ginger, garlic, lemon juice, and ground black pepper. Cook for 1-2 minutes until the sauce is heated through.
5. Return the scallops to the skillet and toss to coat with the sauce.
6. Serve garnished with chopped green onions.

Nutrition Info per Serving:
- Calories: 200
- Protein: 26g
- Carbohydrates: 4g
- Dietary Fiber: 0g
- Sugars: 1g
- Fat: 9g
- Saturated Fat: 1.5g
- Sodium: 420mg

Servings: 4
Cooking Time: 10 minutes

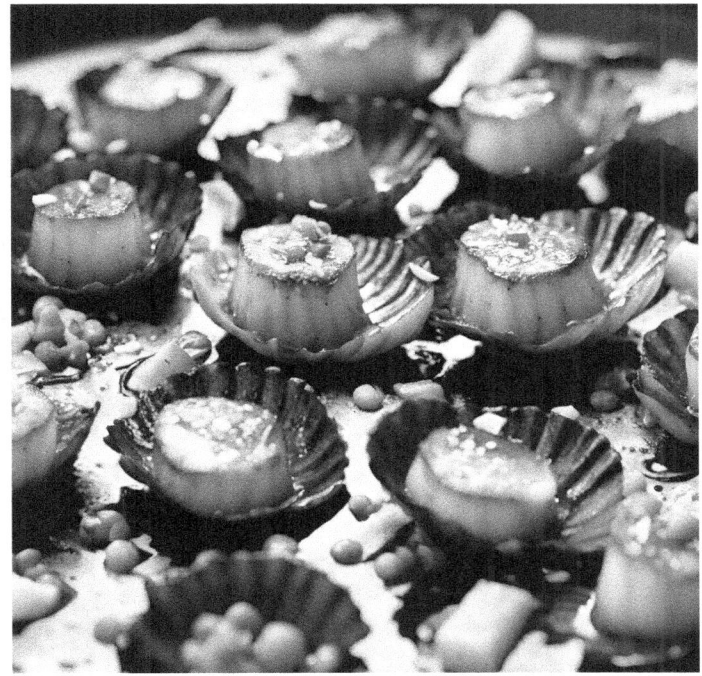

11. Flounder in Parchment

Ingredients:
- 4 flounder fillets (about 6 oz each)
- 2 tbsp olive oil
- 1 lemon, thinly sliced
- 1 zucchini, julienned
- 1 carrot, julienned
- 2 cloves garlic, minced
- 2 tbsp fresh dill, chopped
- 1/2 tsp ground black pepper

Instructions:
1. Preheat the oven to 400°F (200°C).
2. Cut 4 large pieces of parchment paper, each about 15 inches long.
3. Place a flounder fillet in the center of each piece of parchment paper.
4. Drizzle each fillet with olive oil and sprinkle with minced garlic and ground black pepper.
5. Top each fillet with lemon slices, zucchini, and carrot.
6. Sprinkle fresh dill over the vegetables.
7. Fold the parchment paper over the fish and vegetables to create a packet, folding the edges to seal tightly.
8. Place the packets on a baking sheet and bake for 15-20 minutes, or until the fish is cooked through and flakes easily with a fork.
9. Serve the packets unopened for a dramatic presentation.

Nutrition Info per Serving:
- Calories: 220
- Protein: 28g
- Carbohydrates: 6g
- Dietary Fiber: 2g
- Sugars: 3g
- Fat: 10g
- Saturated Fat: 2g
- Sodium: 130mg

Servings: 4
Cooking Time: 20 minutes

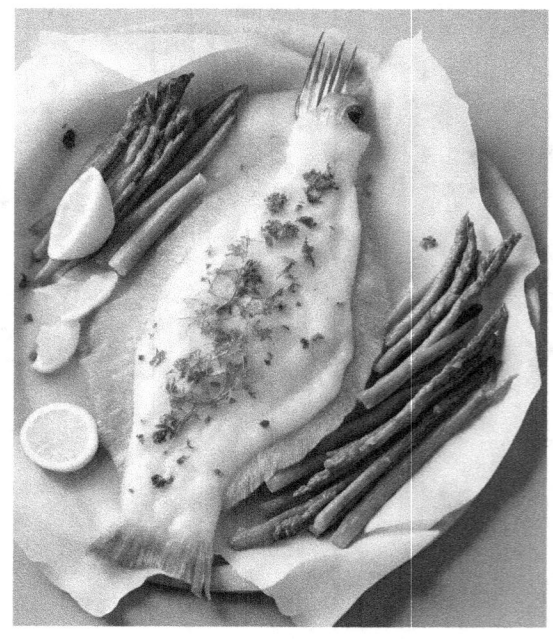

12. Lobster Steamed with Herbs

Ingredients:
- 2 whole lobsters (1.5 lbs each)
- 1 lemon, cut into wedges
- 2 tbsp fresh parsley, chopped
- 2 tbsp fresh tarragon, chopped
- 2 cloves garlic, minced
- 1 tbsp olive oil
- 1/2 tsp ground black pepper

Instructions:
1. Fill a large pot with 2 inches of water and bring to a boil.
2. Add the lemon wedges, garlic, parsley, tarragon, and olive oil to the pot.
3. Place a steaming rack in the pot and place the lobsters on the rack.
4. Cover the pot and steam the lobsters for 12-15 minutes, or until the shells are bright red and the meat is opaque.
5. Remove the lobsters from the pot and let them cool slightly before serving.
6. Serve with the steaming herbs and lemon wedges.

Nutrition Info per Serving:
- Calories: 220
- Protein: 28g
- Carbohydrates: 3g
- Dietary Fiber: 1g
- Sugars: 0g
- Fat: 9g
- Saturated Fat: 2g
- Sodium: 320mg

Servings: 4
Cooking Time: 15 minutes

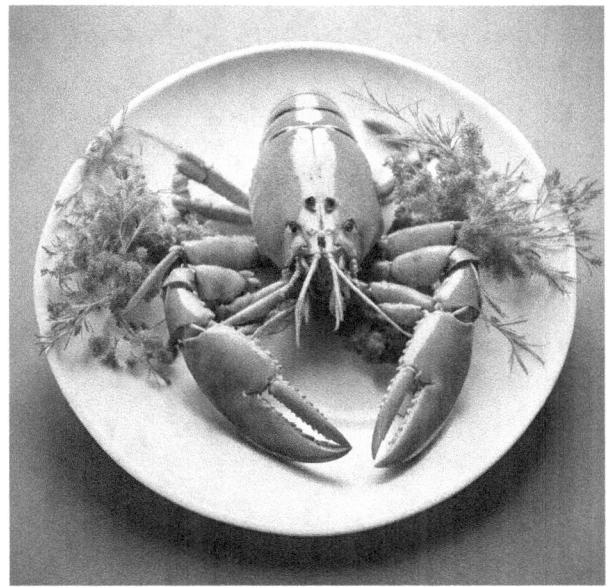

13. Fish Tacos with Cabbage Slaw

Ingredients:
- 1 lb white fish fillets (such as tilapia or cod), cut into strips
- 2 tbsp olive oil
- 1 tbsp lime juice
- 1/2 tsp ground cumin
- 1/2 tsp ground black pepper
- 8 small corn tortillas
- 2 cups shredded cabbage
- 1/2 cup shredded carrots
- 1/4 cup red onion, thinly sliced
- 2 tbsp fresh cilantro, chopped
- 1/4 cup plain Greek yogurt (fat-free)
- 1 tbsp apple cider vinegar

Instructions:
1. In a large bowl, combine the fish strips, olive oil, lime juice, ground cumin, and ground black pepper. Toss to coat.
2. Heat a large skillet over medium-high heat. Add the fish strips and cook for 3-4 minutes per side, or until the fish is cooked through and flakes easily with a fork.
3. In a medium bowl, combine the shredded cabbage, shredded carrots, red onion, and fresh cilantro.
4. In a small bowl, whisk together the Greek yogurt and apple cider vinegar to make the dressing.
5. Pour the dressing over the cabbage mixture and toss to combine.
6. Warm the corn tortillas in a dry skillet or microwave.
7. Assemble the tacos by placing a few strips of fish in each tortilla and topping with the cabbage slaw.
8. Serve immediately.

Nutrition Info per Serving:
- Calories: 210
- Protein: 20g
- Carbohydrates: 20g
- Dietary Fiber: 4g
- Sugars: 3g
- Fat: 8g
- Saturated Fat: 1.5g
- Sodium: 150mg

Servings: 4
Cooking Time: 20 minutes

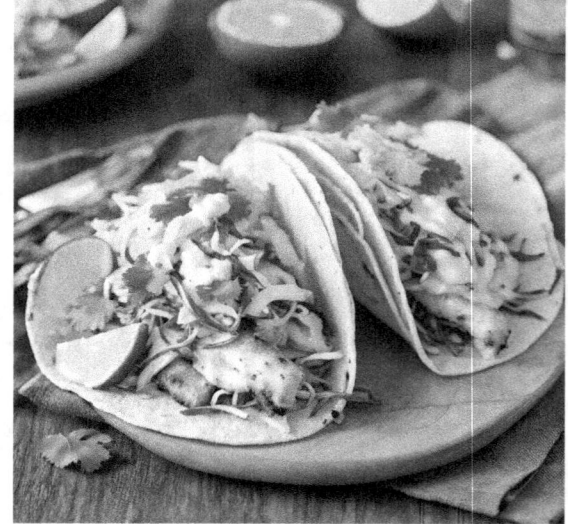

14. Sole Meunière

Ingredients:
- 4 sole fillets (about 6 oz each)
- 1/4 cup whole wheat flour
- 2 tbsp olive oil
- 2 tbsp unsalted butter
- 1 lemon, juiced
- 2 tbsp fresh parsley, chopped
- 1/2 tsp ground black pepper

Instructions:
1. Lightly coat the sole fillets with the whole wheat flour, shaking off any excess.
2. Heat the olive oil in a large skillet over medium heat.
3. Add the fillets to the skillet and cook for 2-3 minutes per side, or until golden brown and cooked through. Remove from the skillet and set aside.
4. In the same skillet, add the butter and let it melt. Add the lemon juice and black pepper, and stir to combine.
5. Return the fillets to the skillet and spoon the sauce over them.
6. Garnish with fresh parsley and serve warm.

Nutrition Info per Serving:
- Calories: 240
- Protein: 28g
- Carbohydrates: 6g
- Dietary Fiber: 1g
- Sugars: 0g
- Fat: 12g
- Saturated Fat: 4g
- Sodium: 150mg

Servings: 4
Cooking Time: 10 minute

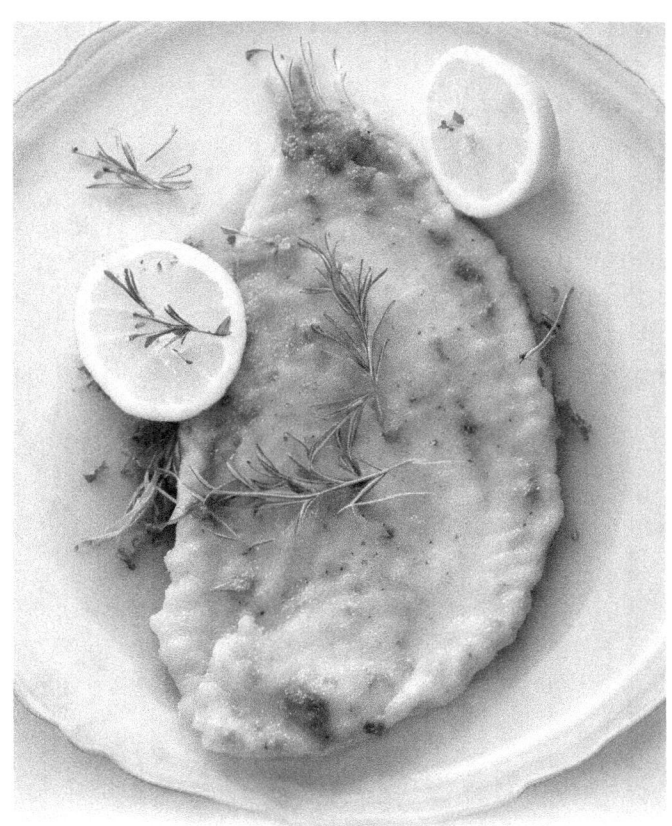

15. Squid Salad with Lime and Cilantro

Ingredients:
- 1 lb squid, cleaned and cut into rings
- 2 tbsp olive oil
- 1/4 cup lime juice
- 1/4 cup red onion, finely chopped
- 1/2 cup cherry tomatoes, halved
- 1 avocado, diced
- 1/2 cup cucumber, diced
- 2 tbsp fresh cilantro, chopped
- 1/2 tsp ground black pepper

Instructions:
1. Bring a large pot of water to a boil. Add the squid rings and cook for 2-3 minutes until tender. Drain and set aside to cool.
2. In a large bowl, whisk together the olive oil, lime juice, and ground black pepper.
3. Add the cooled squid, red onion, cherry tomatoes, avocado, cucumber, and cilantro to the bowl. Toss to combine.
4. Serve chilled.

Nutrition Info per Serving:
- Calories: 220
- Protein: 20g
- Carbohydrates: 10g
- Dietary Fiber: 4g
- Sugars: 2g
- Fat: 12g
- Saturated Fat: 2g
- Sodium: 150mg

Servings: 4
Cooking Time: 10 minutes

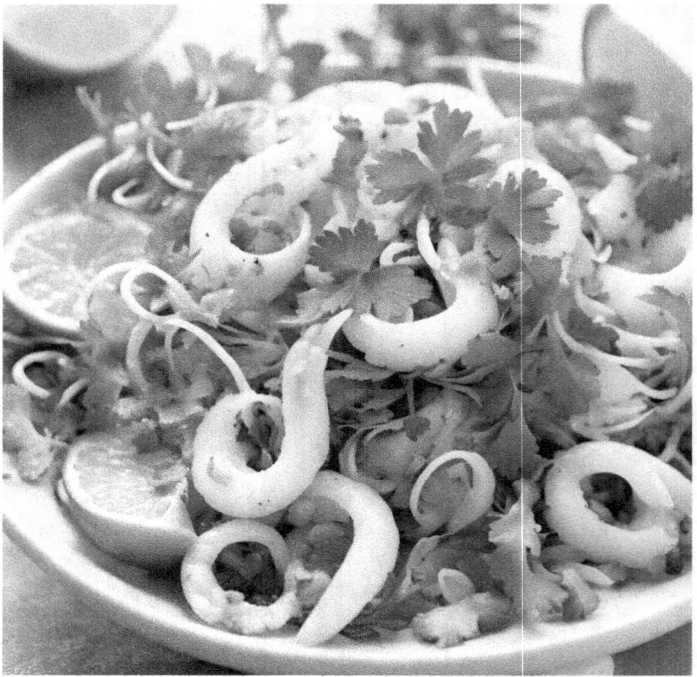

16. Prawn Cocktail with Avocado

Ingredients:
- 1 lb large prawns, peeled and deveined
- 2 avocados, diced
- 1/4 cup red onion, finely chopped
- 1/4 cup cilantro, chopped
- 1 tbsp lime juice
- 1 tbsp olive oil
- 1/2 cup low-sodium tomato sauce
- 1/2 tsp ground black pepper

Instructions:
1. Bring a large pot of water to a boil. Add the prawns and cook for 2-3 minutes, until they are pink and opaque. Drain and let cool.
2. In a large bowl, combine the cooled prawns, diced avocados, red onion, and cilantro.
3. In a small bowl, whisk together the lime juice, olive oil, tomato sauce, and ground black pepper.
4. Pour the dressing over the prawn mixture and toss gently to combine.
5. Serve chilled.

Nutrition Info per Serving:
- Calories: 240
- Protein: 24g
- Carbohydrates: 12g
- Dietary Fiber: 6g
- Sugars: 3g
- Fat: 12g
- Saturated Fat: 2g
- Sodium: 220mg

Servings: 4
Cooking Time: 10 minutes

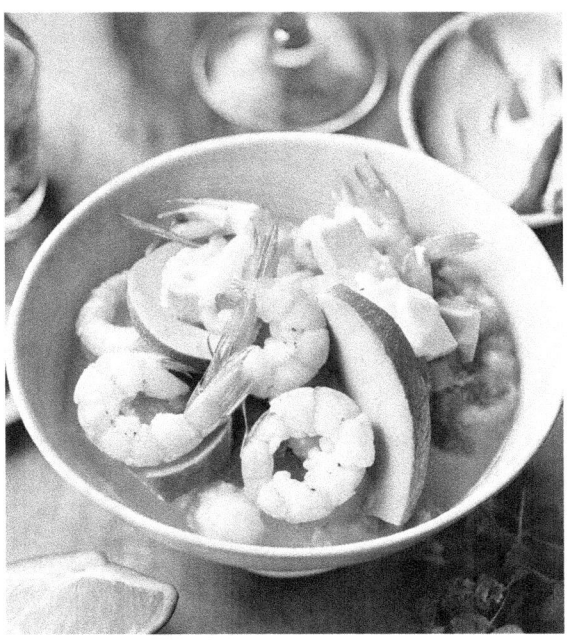

17. Baked Haddock with Tomatoes

Ingredients:
- 4 haddock fillets (about 6 oz each)
- 2 tbsp olive oil
- 1 can (14.5 oz) diced tomatoes, no salt added
- 1 onion, thinly sliced
- 2 cloves garlic, minced
- 1 tsp dried basil
- 1/2 tsp ground black pepper
- 1/4 cup fresh parsley, chopped

Instructions:
1. Preheat the oven to 375°F (190°C).
2. In a baking dish, combine the diced tomatoes, onion, garlic, dried basil, and ground black pepper.
3. Place the haddock fillets on top of the tomato mixture.
4. Drizzle with olive oil.
5. Bake in the preheated oven for 20-25 minutes, or until the fish is cooked through and flakes easily with a fork.
6. Garnish with fresh parsley and serve warm.

Nutrition Info per Serving:
- Calories: 220
- Protein: 30g
- Carbohydrates: 8g
- Dietary Fiber: 2g
- Sugars: 4g
- Fat: 8g
- Saturated Fat: 1.5g
- Sodium: 150mg

Servings: 4
Cooking Time: 25 minutes

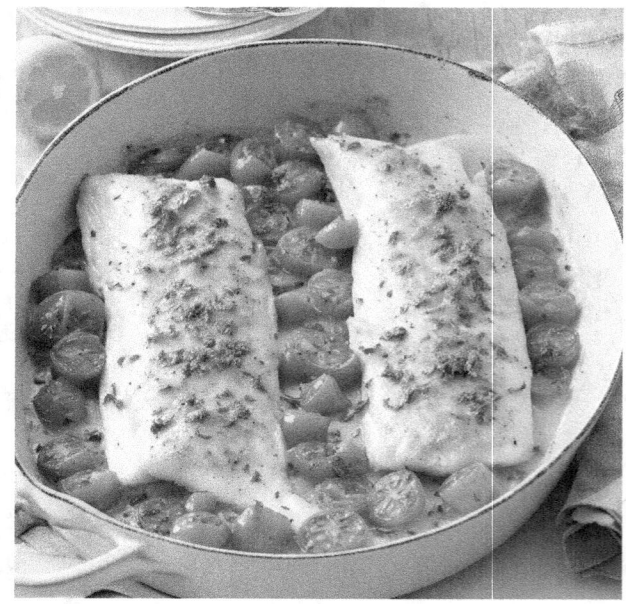

18. Seared Tuna with Sesame Seeds

Ingredients:
- 4 tuna steaks (about 6 oz each)
- 2 tbsp olive oil
- 2 tbsp low-sodium soy sauce
- 1 tbsp fresh ginger, grated
- 1 tbsp sesame seeds
- 1 tbsp fresh lime juice
- 1/2 tsp ground black pepper
- 1 tbsp fresh cilantro, chopped

Instructions:
1. In a small bowl, mix together the olive oil, soy sauce, ginger, lime juice, and ground black pepper.
2. Brush the tuna steaks with the marinade and let sit for 10 minutes.
3. Sprinkle sesame seeds evenly over both sides of the tuna steaks.
4. Heat a non-stick skillet over medium-high heat. Add the tuna steaks and sear for 1-2 minutes per side for rare, or until desired doneness.
5. Remove from the skillet and let rest for a minute before slicing.
6. Garnish with fresh cilantro and serve warm.

Nutrition Info per Serving:
- Calories: 280
- Protein: 34g
- Carbohydrates: 3g
- Dietary Fiber: 1g
- Sugars: 0g
- Fat: 15g
- Saturated Fat: 2g
- Sodium: 180mg

Servings: 4
Cooking Time: 10 minutes

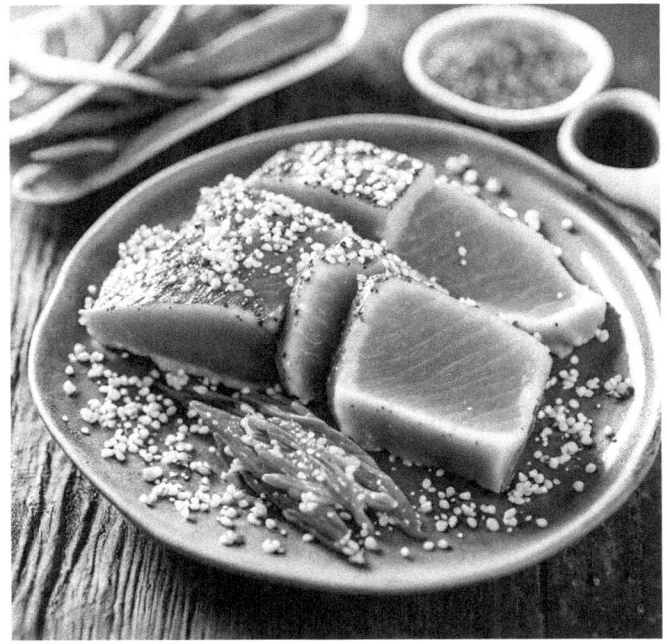

19. Broiled Scallops with Paprika

Ingredients:
- 1 lb sea scallops
- 2 tbsp olive oil
- 1 tsp paprika
- 1/2 tsp ground black pepper
- 1 lemon, cut into wedges
- 2 tbsp fresh parsley, chopped

Instructions:
1. Preheat the broiler.
2. Pat the scallops dry with a paper towel.
3. In a small bowl, mix together the olive oil, paprika, and ground black pepper.
4. Brush the scallops with the olive oil mixture.
5. Place the scallops on a broiler pan and broil for 4-5 minutes per side, or until the scallops are opaque and slightly golden.
6. Serve with lemon wedges and garnished with fresh parsley.

Nutrition Info per Serving:
- Calories: 180
- Protein: 23g
- Carbohydrates: 3g
- Dietary Fiber: 1g
- Sugars: 0g
- Fat: 8g
- Saturated Fat: 1.5g
- Sodium: 190mg

Servings: 4
Cooking Time: 10 minutes

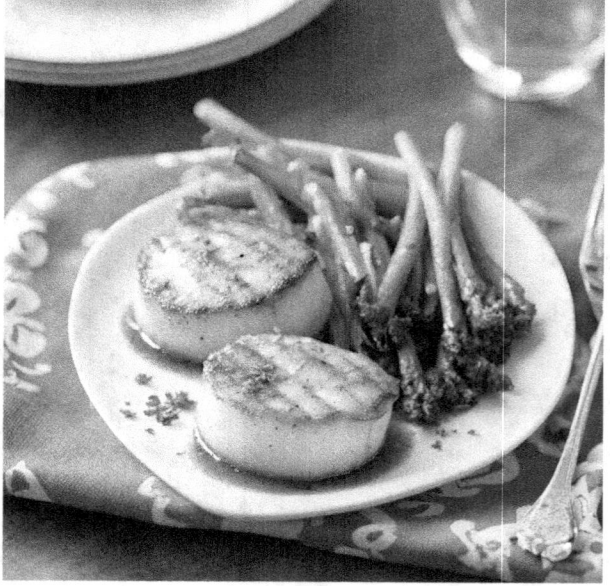

20. Fish Fillet with Parsley Sauce

Ingredients:
- 4 white fish fillets (such as cod or haddock, about 6 oz each)
- 2 tbsp olive oil
- 1/2 cup low-sodium chicken broth
- 1/4 cup fresh parsley, chopped
- 2 cloves garlic, minced
- 1 tbsp lemon juice
- 1/2 tsp ground black pepper

Instructions:
1. Heat the olive oil in a large skillet over medium heat.
2. Add the fish fillets and cook for 3-4 minutes per side, or until the fish is cooked through and flakes easily with a fork. Remove from the skillet and set aside.
3. In the same skillet, add the garlic and cook for 1 minute until fragrant.
4. Stir in the chicken broth, lemon juice, and ground black pepper. Bring to a simmer.
5. Add the parsley and cook for another 2 minutes.
6. Return the fish to the skillet and spoon the sauce over the fillets.
7. Serve warm.

Nutrition Info per Serving:
- Calories: 220
- Protein: 30g
- Carbohydrates: 2g
- Dietary Fiber: 0g
- Sugars: 0g
- Fat: 10g
- Saturated Fat: 1.5g
- Sodium: 180mg

Servings: 4
Cooking Time: 15 minutes

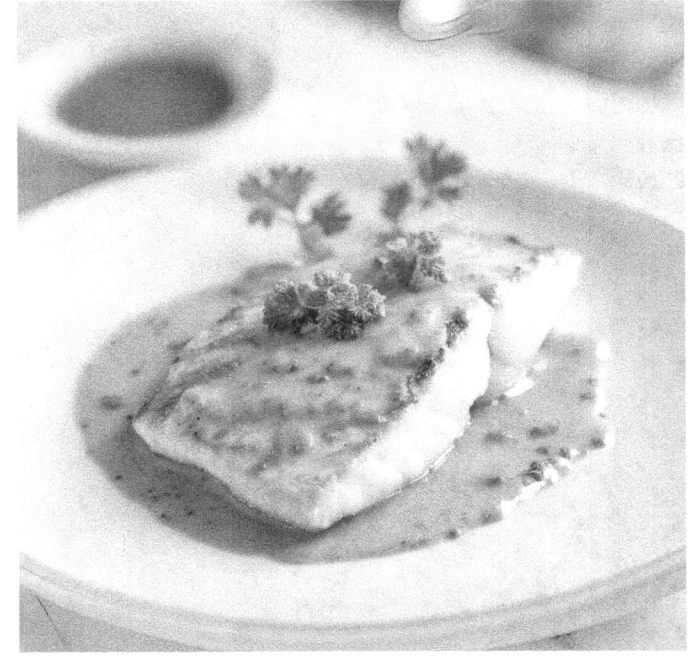

21. Oysters on the Half Shell with Mignonette Sauce

Ingredients:
- 24 fresh oysters, shucked and on the half shell
- 1/4 cup red wine vinegar
- 1 shallot, finely chopped
- 1 tbsp fresh parsley, chopped
- 1 tbsp fresh tarragon, chopped
- 1/2 tsp ground black pepper
- Crushed ice (for serving)

Instructions:
1. In a small bowl, combine the red wine vinegar, chopped shallot, parsley, tarragon, and ground black pepper. Mix well to make the mignonette sauce.
2. Arrange the shucked oysters on a bed of crushed ice.
3. Spoon a small amount of mignonette sauce over each oyster.
4. Serve immediately.

Nutrition Info per Serving:
- Calories: 70
- Protein: 6g
- Carbohydrates: 2g
- Dietary Fiber: 0g
- Sugars: 0g
- Fat: 3g
- Saturated Fat: 0.5g
- Sodium: 160mg

Servings: 4
Cooking Time: 10 minutes

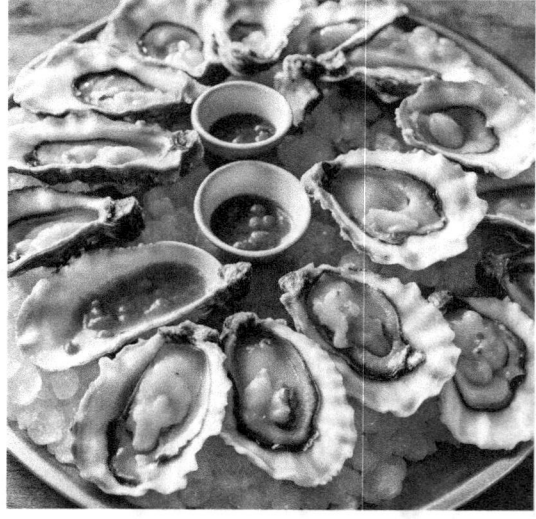

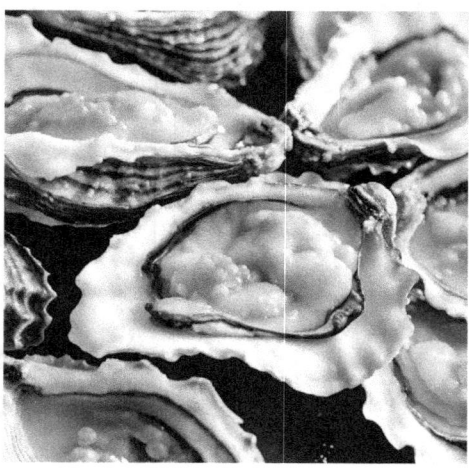

22. Marinated Anchovies with Garlic and Vinegar

Ingredients:
- 1 lb fresh anchovies, cleaned and filleted
- 1/2 cup white wine vinegar
- 2 cloves garlic, thinly sliced
- 2 tbsp olive oil
- 1/4 cup fresh parsley, chopped
- 1/2 tsp ground black pepper
- 1 lemon, sliced

Instructions:
1. In a shallow dish, arrange the anchovy fillets in a single layer.
2. Pour the white wine vinegar over the fillets and sprinkle with sliced garlic.
3. Cover and refrigerate for 1 hour.
4. Remove the anchovies from the vinegar and arrange on a serving plate.
5. Drizzle with olive oil, sprinkle with ground black pepper and fresh parsley.
6. Garnish with lemon slices and serve chilled.

Nutrition Info per Serving:
- Calories: 180
- Protein: 20g
- Carbohydrates: 2g
- Dietary Fiber: 0g
- Sugars: 0g
- Fat: 10g
- Saturated Fat: 2g
- Sodium: 120mg

Servings: 4
Cooking Time: 1 hour (marinating time)

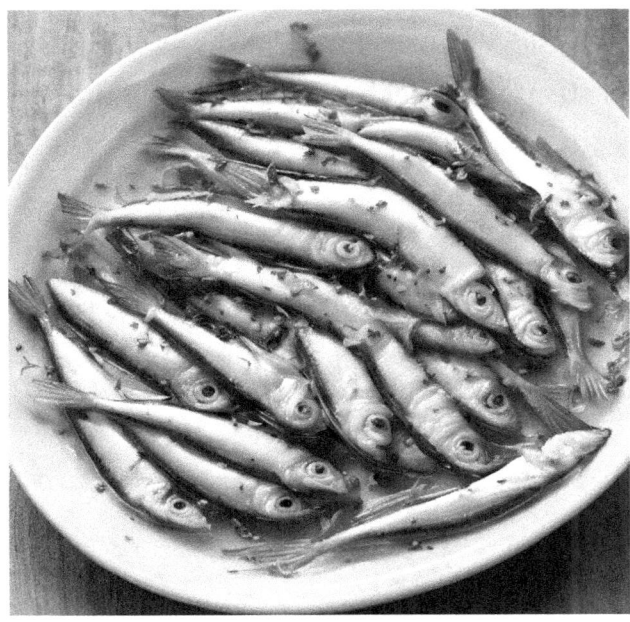

23. Halibut Steaks with Herb Marinade

Ingredients:
- 4 halibut steaks (about 6 oz each)
- 2 tbsp olive oil
- 1 lemon, juiced and zested
- 2 cloves garlic, minced
- 2 tbsp fresh dill, chopped
- 2 tbsp fresh thyme, chopped
- 1/2 tsp ground black pepper

Instructions:
1. In a small bowl, mix together the olive oil, lemon juice, lemon zest, garlic, dill, thyme, and ground black pepper.
2. Place the halibut steaks in a shallow dish and pour the marinade over them, turning to coat evenly.
3. Cover and refrigerate for 30 minutes.
4. Preheat the grill to medium-high heat.
5. Grill the halibut steaks for 5-7 minutes per side, or until the fish is cooked through and flakes easily with a fork.
6. Serve warm.

Nutrition Info per Serving:
- Calories: 250
- Protein: 34g
- Carbohydrates: 2g
- Dietary Fiber: 0g
- Sugars: 0g
- Fat: 11g
- Saturated Fat: 2g
- Sodium: 150mg

Servings: 4
Cooking Time: 40 minutes (including marinating time)

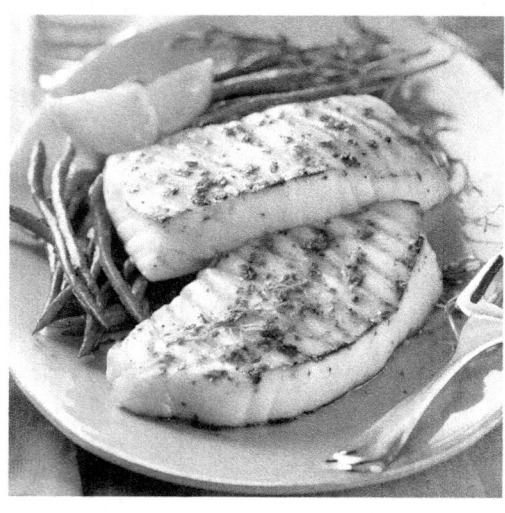

24. Stuffed Squid with Herbed Rice

Ingredients:
- 1 lb squid, cleaned
- 1 cup cooked brown rice
- 2 tbsp olive oil
- 1/4 cup onion, finely chopped
- 2 cloves garlic, minced
- 1/4 cup red bell pepper, finely chopped
- 2 tbsp fresh parsley, chopped
- 1 tbsp fresh basil, chopped
- 1/2 tsp ground black pepper

Instructions:
1. Preheat the oven to 375°F (190°C).
2. In a skillet, heat 1 tbsp olive oil over medium heat. Add the onion, garlic, and red bell pepper. Cook until softened, about 3-4 minutes.
3. Stir in the cooked rice, parsley, basil, and ground black pepper. Cook for another 2 minutes.
4. Stuff the squid with the rice mixture and secure with toothpicks.
5. Place the stuffed squid in a baking dish and drizzle with the remaining olive oil.
6. Bake in the preheated oven for 20-25 minutes, or until the squid is tender.
7. Serve warm.

Nutrition Info per Serving:
- Calories: 220
- Protein: 24g
- Carbohydrates: 18g
- Dietary Fiber: 3g
- Sugars: 2g
- Fat: 8g
- Saturated Fat: 1.5g
- Sodium: 200mg

Servings: 4
Cooking Time: 35 minutes

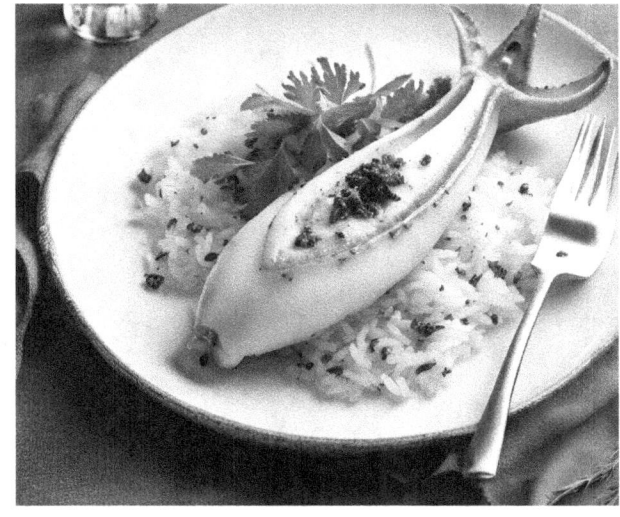

25. Sardines Grilled with Lemon

Ingredients:
- 1 lb fresh sardines, cleaned
- 2 tbsp olive oil
- 1 lemon, sliced
- 1 tbsp fresh parsley, chopped
- 1/2 tsp ground black pepper

Instructions:
1. Preheat the grill to medium-high heat.
2. Brush the sardines with olive oil and sprinkle with ground black pepper.
3. Place the sardines on the grill and cook for 3-4 minutes per side, or until cooked through.
4. Arrange the grilled sardines on a serving plate and garnish with lemon slices and fresh parsley.
5. Serve warm.

Nutrition Info per Serving:
- Calories: 200
- Protein: 22g
- Carbohydrates: 2g
- Dietary Fiber: 0g
- Sugars: 0g
- Fat: 12g
- Saturated Fat: 2.5g
- Sodium: 180mg

Servings: 4
Cooking Time: 10 minutes

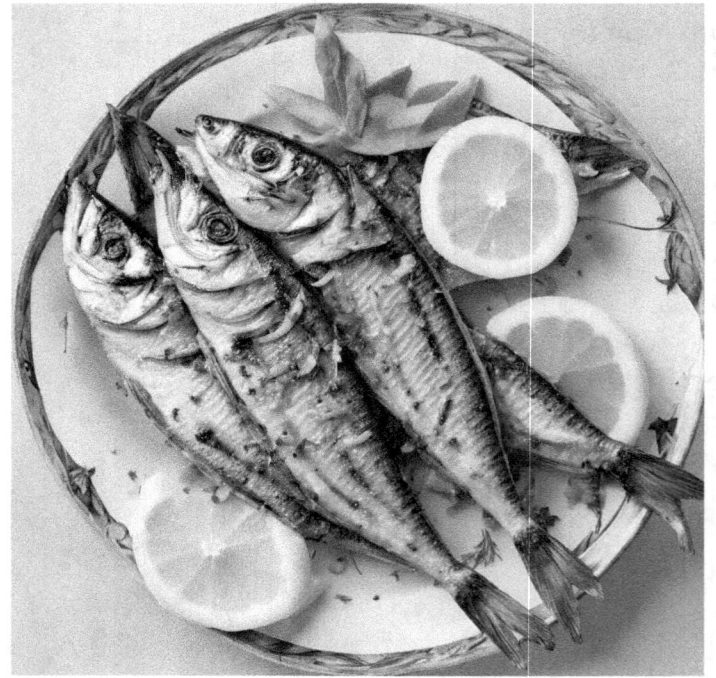

26. Panko-Crusted Tilapia

Ingredients:
- 4 tilapia fillets (about 6 oz each)
- 1 cup whole wheat panko breadcrumbs
- 1/4 cup grated Parmesan cheese
- 2 tbsp fresh parsley, chopped
- 1/2 tsp ground black pepper
- 2 tbsp olive oil
- 1 lemon, cut into wedges

Instructions:
1. Preheat the oven to 400°F (200°C). Line a baking sheet with parchment paper.
2. In a shallow dish, mix together the panko breadcrumbs, Parmesan cheese, parsley, and ground black pepper.
3. Brush each tilapia fillet with olive oil, then press into the breadcrumb mixture to coat evenly.
4. Place the coated fillets on the prepared baking sheet.
5. Bake in the preheated oven for 12-15 minutes, or until the fish is cooked through and the crust is golden brown.
6. Serve with lemon wedges.

Nutrition Info per Serving:
- Calories: 270
- Protein: 30g
- Carbohydrates: 10g
- Dietary Fiber: 2g
- Sugars: 0g
- Fat: 12g
- Saturated Fat: 3g
- Sodium: 200mg

Servings: 4
Cooking Time: 15 minutes

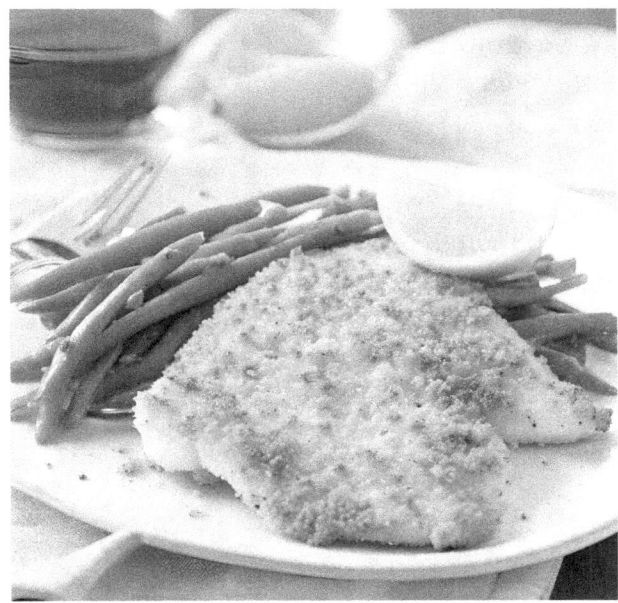

27. Mackerel in Tomato Sauce

Ingredients:
- 4 mackerel fillets (about 6 oz each)
- 2 tbsp olive oil
- 1 onion, chopped
- 2 cloves garlic, minced
- 1 can (14.5 oz) diced tomatoes, no salt added
- 1 tsp dried oregano
- 1/2 tsp ground black pepper
- 1/4 cup fresh basil, chopped

Instructions:
1. Preheat the oven to 375°F (190°C).
2. Heat the olive oil in a skillet over medium heat. Add the onion and garlic, and cook until softened, about 3-4 minutes.
3. Stir in the diced tomatoes, dried oregano, and ground black pepper. Simmer for 5 minutes.
4. Place the mackerel fillets in a baking dish and pour the tomato sauce over them.
5. Bake in the preheated oven for 20-25 minutes, or until the fish is cooked through and flakes easily with a fork.
6. Garnish with fresh basil and serve warm.

Nutrition Info per Serving:
- Calories: 250
- Protein: 30g
- Carbohydrates: 6g
- Dietary Fiber: 2g
- Sugars: 3g
- Fat: 12g
- Saturated Fat: 2g
- Sodium: 150mg

Servings: 4
Cooking Time: 30 minutes

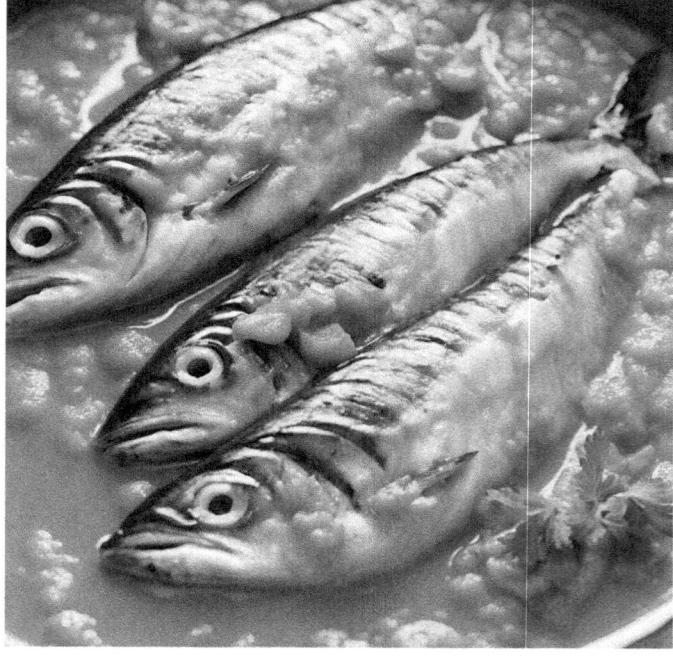

28. Peppered Mackerel on Rye

Ingredients:
- 4 smoked mackerel fillets (about 6 oz each)
- 4 slices rye bread
- 1 tbsp Dijon mustard
- 1 tbsp olive oil
- 1/4 cup red onion, thinly sliced
- 1/4 cup fresh parsley, chopped
- 1/2 tsp ground black pepper

Instructions:
1. Toast the rye bread slices until golden brown.
2. Spread Dijon mustard evenly on each slice of toast.
3. Top each slice with a smoked mackerel fillet.
4. Drizzle with olive oil and sprinkle with ground black pepper.
5. Garnish with red onion slices and fresh parsley.
6. Serve immediately.

Nutrition Info per Serving:
- Calories: 300
- Protein: 25g
- Carbohydrates: 20g
- Dietary Fiber: 4g
- Sugars: 2g
- Fat: 15g
- Saturated Fat: 3g
- Sodium: 250mg

Servings: 4
Cooking Time: 10 minutes

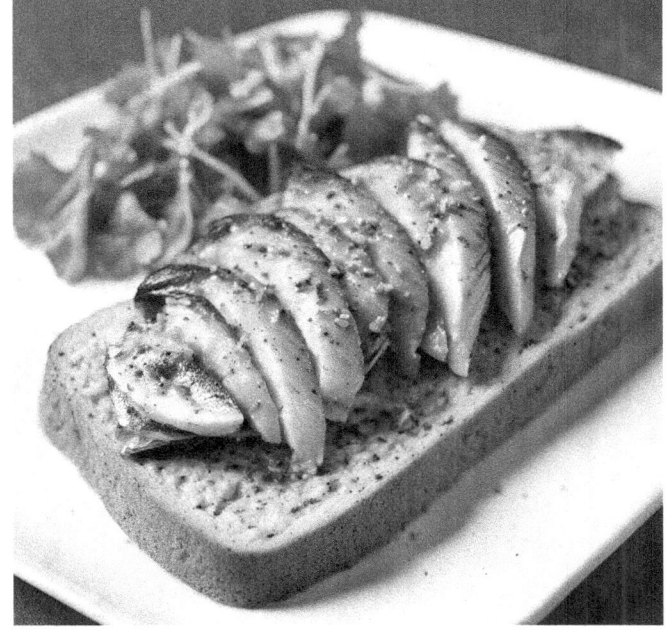

29. Grilled Eel with Teriyaki Sauce

Ingredients:
- 4 eel fillets (about 6 oz each)
- 2 tbsp olive oil
- 1/4 cup low-sodium soy sauce
- 2 tbsp mirin (Japanese sweet rice wine)
- 1 tbsp honey
- 1 tbsp fresh ginger, grated
- 1/2 tsp ground black pepper
- 2 tbsp sesame seeds
- 2 green onions, chopped

Instructions:
1. In a small bowl, mix together the soy sauce, mirin, honey, ginger, and ground black pepper.
2. Marinate the eel fillets in the sauce for 30 minutes.
3. Preheat the grill to medium-high heat.
4. Brush the eel fillets with olive oil and grill for 4-5 minutes per side, or until cooked through and slightly charred.
5. Sprinkle with sesame seeds and garnish with green onions.
6. Serve warm.

Nutrition Info per Serving:
- Calories: 280
- Protein: 25g
- Carbohydrates: 8g
- Dietary Fiber: 1g
- Sugars: 5g
- Fat: 15g
- Saturated Fat: 3g
- Sodium: 300mg

Servings: 4
Cooking Time: 40 minutes (including marinating time)

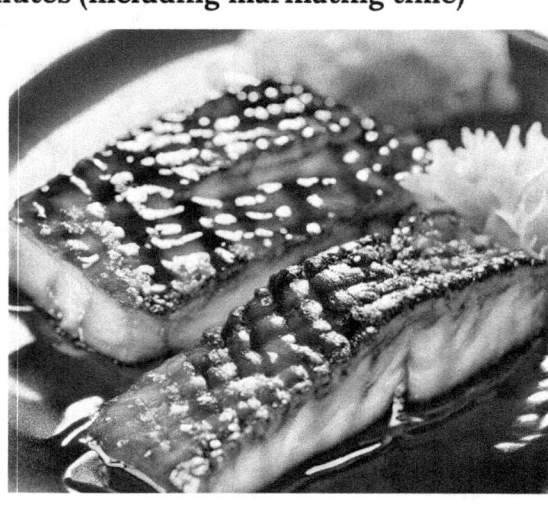

30. Linguine with Clams

Ingredients:
- 1 lb fresh clams, scrubbed
- 8 oz whole wheat linguine
- 2 tbsp olive oil
- 3 cloves garlic, minced
- 1/2 cup white wine (optional, can substitute with more broth)
- 1 cup low-sodium chicken broth
- 1/2 tsp ground black pepper
- 1/4 cup fresh parsley, chopped
- 1 lemon, cut into wedges

Instructions:
1. Cook the linguine according to package instructions until al dente. Drain and set aside.
2. In a large pot, heat the olive oil over medium heat. Add the garlic and cook for 1 minute until fragrant.
3. Add the white wine (if using) and chicken broth, and bring to a simmer.
4. Add the clams and cover the pot. Cook for 5-7 minutes, or until the clams open. Discard any clams that do not open.
5. Stir in the cooked linguine, ground black pepper, and fresh parsley.
6. Serve with lemon wedges.

Nutrition Info per Serving:
- Calories: 300
- Protein: 20g
- Carbohydrates: 40g
- Dietary Fiber: 6g
- Sugars: 2g
- Fat: 8g
- Saturated Fat: 1.5g
- Sodium: 400mg

Servings: 4
Cooking Time: 20 minutes

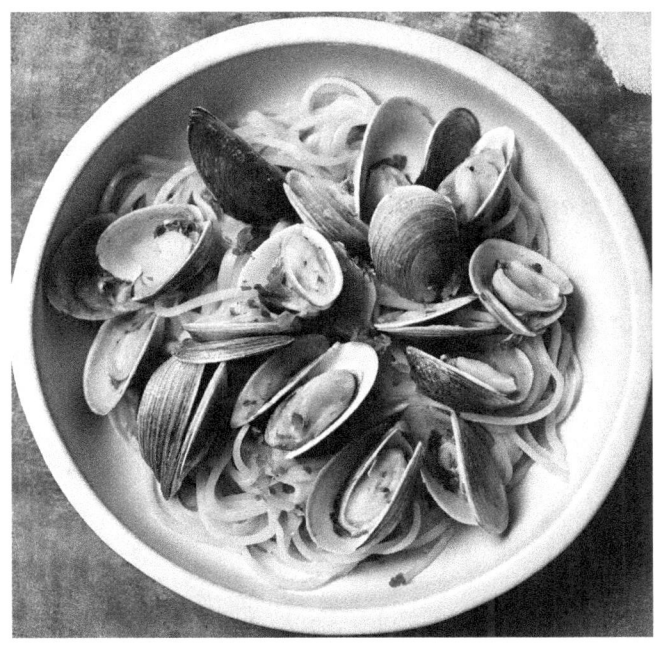

31. Monkfish with Saffron Broth

Ingredients:
- 4 monkfish fillets (about 6 oz each)
- 2 tbsp olive oil
- 1 onion, finely chopped
- 2 cloves garlic, minced
- 1 cup low-sodium chicken broth
- 1/2 cup white wine (optional, can substitute with more broth)
- 1/4 tsp saffron threads
- 1/2 tsp ground black pepper
- 1/4 cup fresh parsley, chopped

Instructions:
1. Heat the olive oil in a large skillet over medium heat. Add the onion and garlic, and cook until softened, about 3-4 minutes.
2. Stir in the chicken broth, white wine (if using), saffron, and ground black pepper. Bring to a simmer.
3. Add the monkfish fillets to the skillet and cover. Simmer for 10-12 minutes, or until the fish is cooked through and flakes easily with a fork.
4. Remove the fish from the skillet and keep warm.
5. Continue to simmer the broth for another 2-3 minutes until slightly reduced.
6. Serve the monkfish with the saffron broth, garnished with fresh parsley.

Nutrition Info per Serving:
- Calories: 280
- Protein: 35g
- Carbohydrates: 4g
- Dietary Fiber: 1g
- Sugars: 1g
- Fat: 12g
- Saturated Fat: 2.5g
- Sodium: 300mg

Servings: 4
Cooking Time: 20 minutes

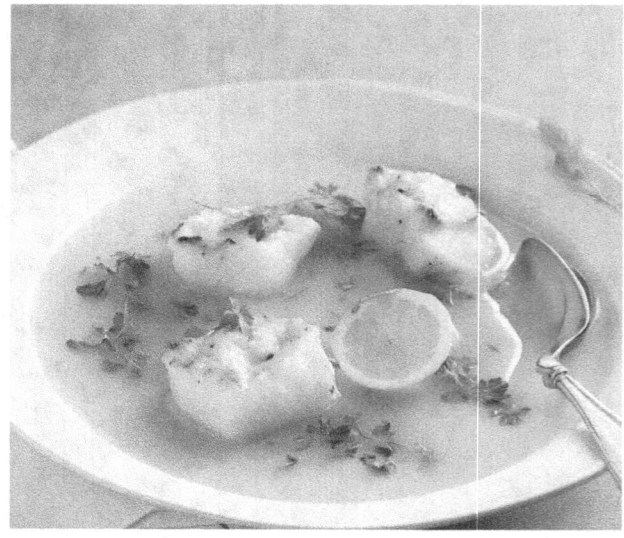

Soup and Stew Recipes

1. Carrot and Ginger Soup
Ingredients:
- 1 tbsp olive oil
- 1 onion, chopped
- 1 lb carrots, peeled and chopped
- 2 cloves garlic, minced
- 1 tbsp fresh ginger, grated
- 4 cups low-sodium vegetable broth
- 1/2 tsp ground black pepper
- 1/4 cup fresh parsley, chopped (optional for garnish)

Instructions:
1. Heat the olive oil in a large pot over medium heat.
2. Add the onion and cook until softened, about 3-4 minutes.
3. Add the garlic and ginger, and cook for another 1-2 minutes.
4. Stir in the chopped carrots and cook for 5 minutes.
5. Pour in the vegetable broth and ground black pepper, bring to a boil.
6. Reduce heat and simmer for 20-25 minutes, until the carrots are tender.
7. Use an immersion blender to puree the soup until smooth (or transfer to a blender in batches).
8. Serve warm, garnished with fresh parsley if desired.

Nutrition Info per Serving:
- Calories: 150
- Protein: 2g
- Carbohydrates: 20g
- Dietary Fiber: 5g
- Sugars: 10g
- Fat: 7g
- Saturated Fat: 1g
- Sodium: 150mg

Servings: 4
Cooking Time: 35 minutes

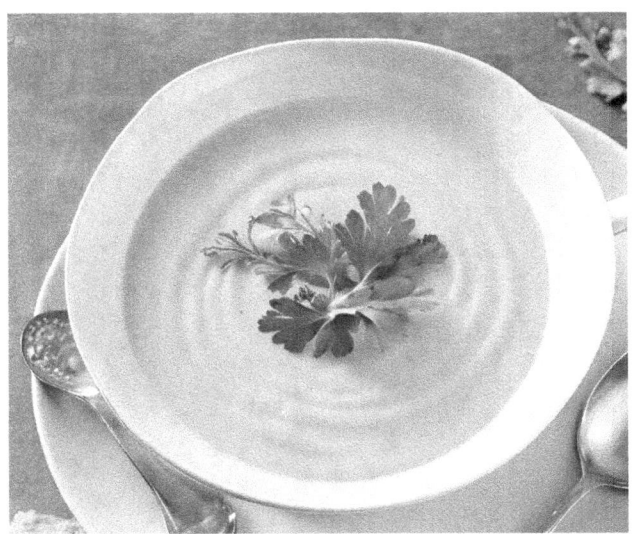

2. Lentil and Spinach Soup

Ingredients:
- 1 tbsp olive oil
- 1 onion, chopped
- 2 cloves garlic, minced
- 1 cup dried lentils, rinsed
- 1 carrot, chopped
- 1 celery stalk, chopped
- 4 cups low-sodium vegetable broth
- 1/2 tsp ground cumin
- 1/2 tsp ground black pepper
- 4 cups fresh spinach, chopped
- 1/4 cup fresh cilantro, chopped (optional for garnish)

Instructions:
1. Heat the olive oil in a large pot over medium heat.
2. Add the onion and cook until softened, about 3-4 minutes.
3. Add the garlic and cook for another 1-2 minutes.
4. Stir in the lentils, carrot, and celery, and cook for 5 minutes.
5. Pour in the vegetable broth, ground cumin, and ground black pepper. Bring to a boil.
6. Reduce heat and simmer for 25-30 minutes, until the lentils are tender.
7. Stir in the chopped spinach and cook for another 2-3 minutes until wilted.
8. Serve warm, garnished with fresh cilantro if desired.

Nutrition Info per Serving:
- Calories: 200
- Protein: 12g
- Carbohydrates: 30g
- Dietary Fiber: 12g
- Sugars: 5g
- Fat: 6g
- Saturated Fat: 1g
- Sodium: 180mg

Servings: 4
Cooking Time: 40 minutes

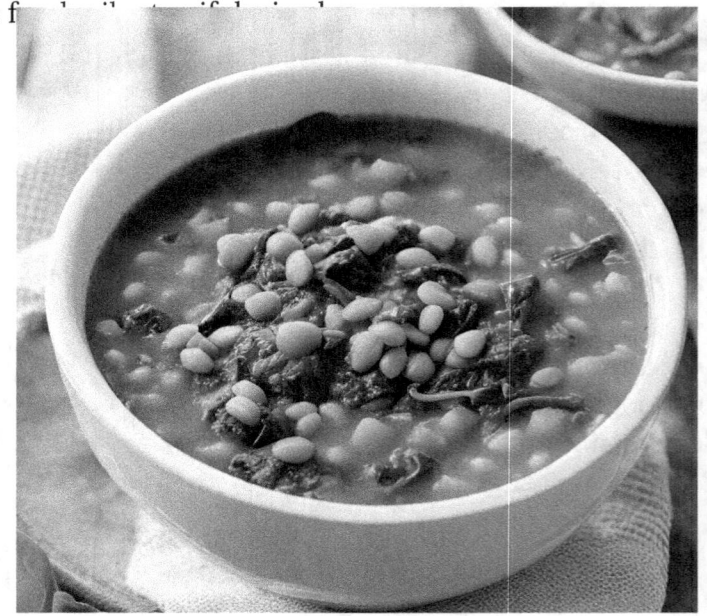

3. Chickpea and Vegetable Stew

Ingredients:
- 1 tbsp olive oil
- 1 onion, chopped
- 2 cloves garlic, minced
- 1 carrot, chopped
- 1 zucchini, chopped
- 1 red bell pepper, chopped
- 1 can (14.5 oz) diced tomatoes, no salt added
- 1 can (15 oz) chickpeas, drained and rinsed
- 4 cups low-sodium vegetable broth
- 1 tsp ground cumin
- 1/2 tsp ground black pepper
- 1/4 cup fresh parsley, chopped (optional for garnish)

Instructions:
1. Heat the olive oil in a large pot over medium heat.
2. Add the onion and cook until softened, about 3-4 minutes.
3. Add the garlic and cook for another 1-2 minutes.
4. Stir in the carrot, zucchini, and red bell pepper, and cook for 5 minutes.
5. Pour in the diced tomatoes, chickpeas, vegetable broth, ground cumin, and ground black pepper. Bring to a boil.
6. Reduce heat and simmer for 25-30 minutes, until the vegetables are tender.
7. Serve warm, garnished with fresh parsley if desired.

Nutrition Info per Serving:
- Calories: 220
- Protein: 8g
- Carbohydrates: 35g
- Dietary Fiber: 10g
- Sugars: 7g
- Fat: 7g
- Saturated Fat: 1g
- Sodium: 200mg

Servings: 4
Cooking Time: 40 minutes

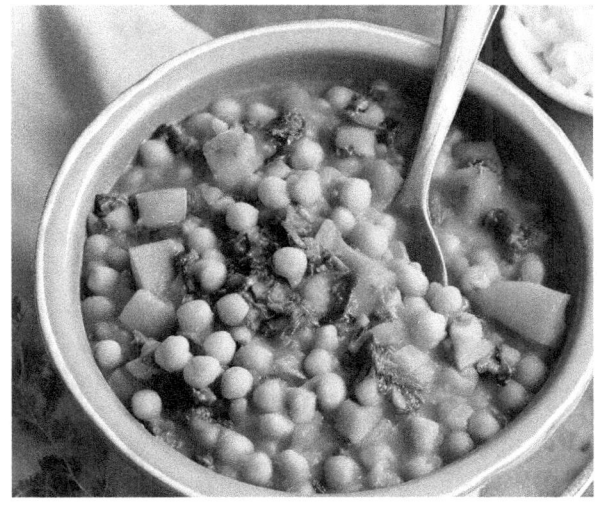

4. Split Pea Soup

Ingredients:
- 1 tbsp olive oil
- 1 onion, chopped
- 2 cloves garlic, minced
- 2 carrots, chopped
- 2 celery stalks, chopped
- 1 cup dried split peas, rinsed
- 4 cups low-sodium vegetable broth
- 1/2 tsp dried thyme
- 1/2 tsp ground black pepper
- 1 bay leaf
- 1/4 cup fresh parsley, chopped (optional for garnish)

Instructions:
1. Heat the olive oil in a large pot over medium heat.
2. Add the onion and cook until softened, about 3-4 minutes.
3. Add the garlic and cook for another 1-2 minutes.
4. Stir in the carrots, celery, and split peas, and cook for 5 minutes.
5. Pour in the vegetable broth, dried thyme, ground black pepper, and bay leaf. Bring to a boil.
6. Reduce heat and simmer for 45-50 minutes, until the peas are tender.
7. Remove the bay leaf and use an immersion blender to puree the soup until smooth (or transfer to a blender in batches).
8. Serve warm, garnished with fresh parsley if desired.

Nutrition Info per Serving:
- Calories: 210
- Protein: 11g
- Carbohydrates: 38g
- Dietary Fiber: 15g
- Sugars: 7g
- Fat: 4g
- Saturated Fat: 0.5g
- Sodium: 180mg

Servings: 4
Cooking Time: 55 minutes

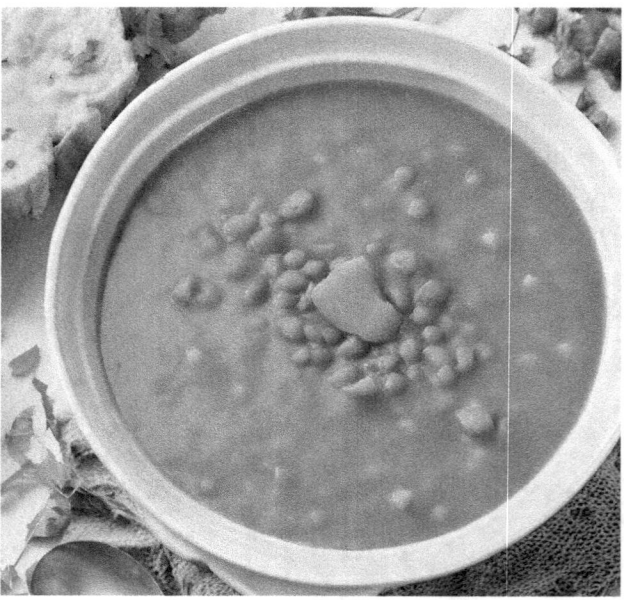

5. Pumpkin Soup

Ingredients:
- 1 tbsp olive oil
- 1 onion, chopped
- 2 cloves garlic, minced
- 4 cups pumpkin, peeled and chopped
- 4 cups low-sodium vegetable broth
- 1/2 tsp ground ginger
- 1/2 tsp ground black pepper
- 1/4 tsp ground nutmeg
- 1/2 cup skim milk (or dairy-free alternative)
- 1/4 cup fresh chives, chopped (optional for garnish)

Instructions:
1. Heat the olive oil in a large pot over medium heat.
2. Add the onion and cook until softened, about 3-4 minutes.
3. Add the garlic and cook for another 1-2 minutes.
4. Stir in the chopped pumpkin and cook for 5 minutes.
5. Pour in the vegetable broth, ground ginger, ground black pepper, and ground nutmeg. Bring to a boil.
6. Reduce heat and simmer for 20-25 minutes, until the pumpkin is tender.
7. Use an immersion blender to puree the soup until smooth (or transfer to a blender in batches).
8. Stir in the skim milk and heat through.
9. Serve warm, garnished with fresh chives if desired.

Nutrition Info per Serving:
- Calories: 160
- Protein: 3g
- Carbohydrates: 25g
- Dietary Fiber: 5g
- Sugars: 10g
- Fat: 6g
- Saturated Fat: 1g
- Sodium: 160mg

Servings: 4
Cooking Time: 30 minutes

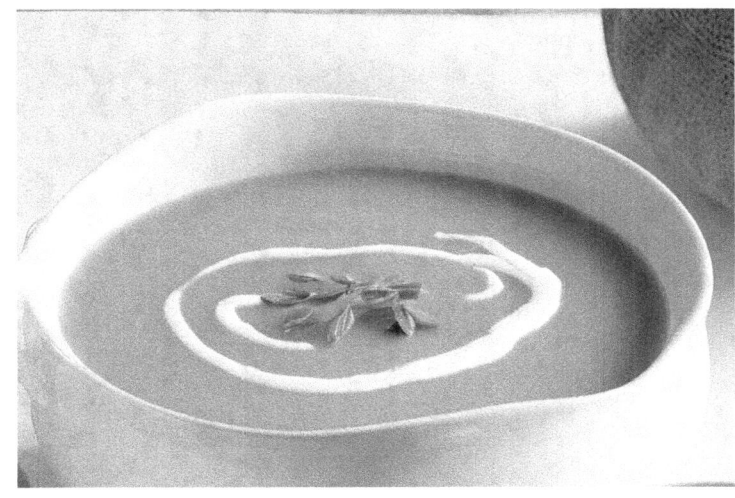

6. Bean and Barley Soup

Ingredients:
- 1 tbsp olive oil
- 1 onion, chopped
- 2 cloves garlic, minced
- 1 carrot, chopped
- 1 celery stalk, chopped
- 1/2 cup pearl barley
- 1 can (15 oz) white beans, drained and rinsed
- 4 cups low-sodium vegetable broth
- 1/2 tsp dried thyme
- 1/2 tsp ground black pepper
- 1 bay leaf
- 1/4 cup fresh parsley, chopped (optional for garnish)

Instructions:
1. Heat the olive oil in a large pot over medium heat.
2. Add the onion and cook until softened, about 3-4 minutes.
3. Add the garlic and cook for another 1-2 minutes.
4. Stir in the carrot, celery, and barley. Cook for 5 minutes.
5. Pour in the vegetable broth, beans, dried thyme, ground black pepper, and bay leaf. Bring to a boil.
6. Reduce heat and simmer for 40-45 minutes, until the barley is tender.
7. Remove the bay leaf and serve warm, garnished with fresh parsley if desired.

Nutrition Info per Serving:
- Calories: 220
- Protein: 8g
- Carbohydrates: 40g
- Dietary Fiber: 10g
- Sugars: 5g
- Fat: 4g
- Saturated Fat: 0.5g
- Sodium: 180mg

Servings: 4
Cooking Time: 50 minutes

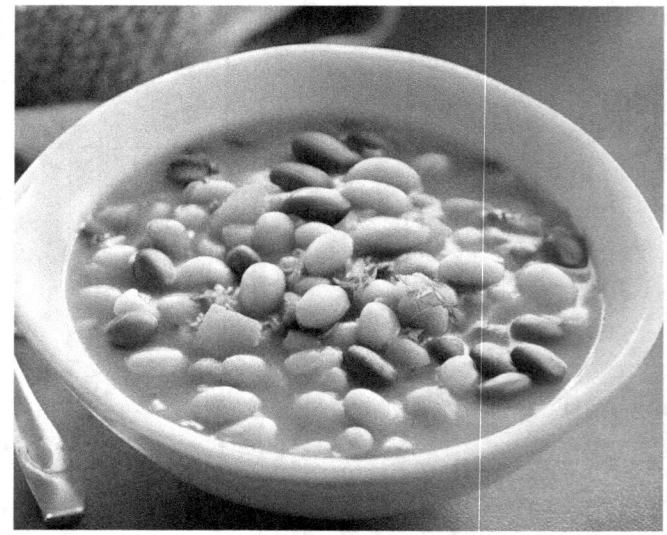

7. Cabbage Soup
Ingredients:
- 1 tbsp olive oil
- 1 onion, chopped
- 2 cloves garlic, minced
- 4 cups cabbage, shredded
- 2 carrots, chopped
- 2 celery stalks, chopped
- 1 can (14.5 oz) diced tomatoes, no salt added
- 4 cups low-sodium vegetable broth
- 1/2 tsp dried thyme
- 1/2 tsp ground black pepper
- 1 bay leaf
- 1/4 cup fresh dill, chopped (optional for garnish)

Instructions:
1. Heat the olive oil in a large pot over medium heat.
2. Add the onion and cook until softened, about 3-4 minutes.
3. Add the garlic and cook for another 1-2 minutes.
4. Stir in the cabbage, carrots, and celery. Cook for 5 minutes.
5. Pour in the diced tomatoes, vegetable broth, dried thyme, ground black pepper, and bay leaf. Bring to a boil.
6. Reduce heat and simmer for 30-35 minutes, until the vegetables are tender.
7. Remove the bay leaf and serve warm, garnished with fresh dill if desired.

Nutrition Info per Serving:
- Calories: 140
- Protein: 4g
- Carbohydrates: 28g
- Dietary Fiber: 8g
- Sugars: 10g
- Fat: 3g
- Saturated Fat: 0.5g
- Sodium: 180mg

Servings: 4
Cooking Time: 40 minutes

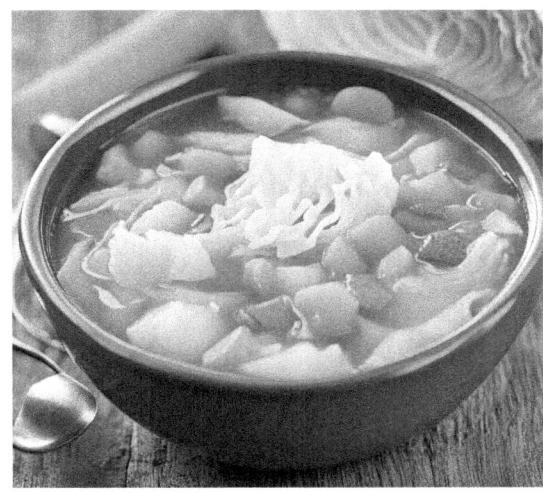

8. Vegetable Minestrone

Ingredients:
- 1 tbsp olive oil
- 1 onion, chopped
- 2 cloves garlic, minced
- 2 carrots, chopped
- 2 celery stalks, chopped
- 1 zucchini, chopped
- 1 can (14.5 oz) diced tomatoes, no salt added
- 4 cups low-sodium vegetable broth
- 1 can (15 oz) kidney beans, drained and rinsed
- 1/2 cup whole wheat pasta (small shapes)
- 1 tsp dried oregano
- 1/2 tsp ground black pepper
- 1/4 cup fresh basil, chopped (optional for garnish)

Instructions:
1. Heat the olive oil in a large pot over medium heat.
2. Add the onion and cook until softened, about 3-4 minutes.
3. Add the garlic and cook for another 1-2 minutes.
4. Stir in the carrots, celery, and zucchini. Cook for 5 minutes.
5. Pour in the diced tomatoes, vegetable broth, and beans. Bring to a boil.
6. Stir in the pasta, dried oregano, and ground black pepper.
7. Reduce heat and simmer for 10-12 minutes, until the pasta and vegetables are tender.
8. Serve warm, garnished with fresh basil if desired.

Nutrition Info per Serving:
- Calories: 220
- Protein: 8g
- Carbohydrates: 40g
- Dietary Fiber: 10g
- Sugars: 7g
- Fat: 5g
- Saturated Fat: 1g
- Sodium: 180mg

Servings: 4
Cooking Time: 30 minutes

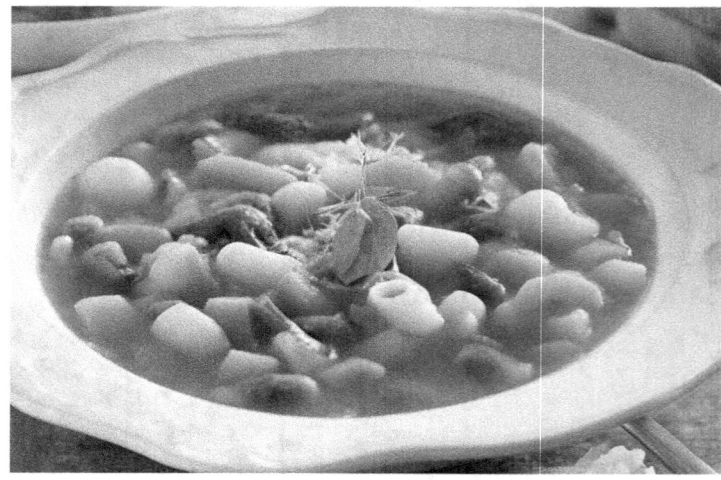

9. Sweet Potato and Lentil Soup

Ingredients:
- 1 tbsp olive oil
- 1 onion, chopped
- 2 cloves garlic, minced
- 1 cup dried red lentils, rinsed
- 2 sweet potatoes, peeled and chopped
- 4 cups low-sodium vegetable broth
- 1 tsp ground cumin
- 1/2 tsp ground black pepper
- 1/4 tsp ground cinnamon
- 1/4 cup fresh cilantro, chopped (optional for garnish)

Instructions:
1. Heat the olive oil in a large pot over medium heat.
2. Add the onion and cook until softened, about 3-4 minutes.
3. Add the garlic and cook for another 1-2 minutes.
4. Stir in the lentils and sweet potatoes. Cook for 5 minutes.
5. Pour in the vegetable broth, ground cumin, ground black pepper, and ground cinnamon. Bring to a boil.
6. Reduce heat and simmer for 25-30 minutes, until the lentils and sweet potatoes are tender.
7. Use an immersion blender to puree the soup until smooth (or transfer to a blender in batches).
8. Serve warm, garnished with fresh cilantro if desired.

Nutrition Info per Serving:
- Calories: 240
- Protein: 10g
- Carbohydrates: 45g
- Dietary Fiber: 12g
- Sugars: 10g
- Fat: 4g
- Saturated Fat: 0.5g
- Sodium: 180mg

Servings: 4
Cooking Time: 35 minutes

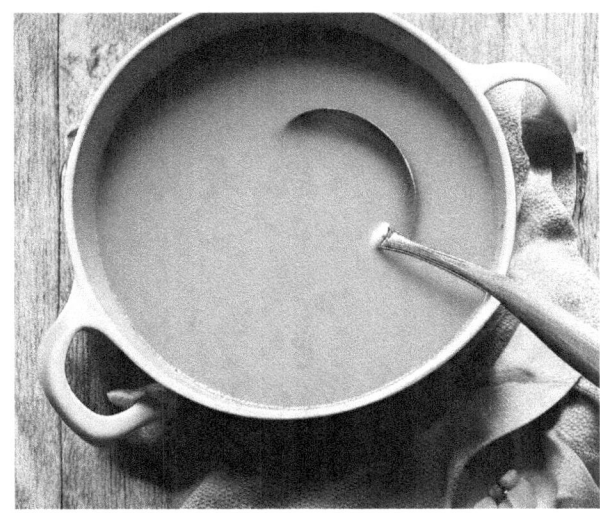

10. Mushroom and Leek Soup

Ingredients:
- 1 tbsp olive oil
- 2 leeks, cleaned and sliced
- 2 cloves garlic, minced
- 1 lb mushrooms, sliced
- 4 cups low-sodium vegetable broth
- 1/2 tsp dried thyme
- 1/2 tsp ground black pepper
- 1/2 cup skim milk (or dairy-free alternative)
- 1/4 cup fresh chives, chopped (optional for garnish)

Instructions:
1. Heat the olive oil in a large pot over medium heat.
2. Add the leeks and cook until softened, about 3-4 minutes.
3. Add the garlic and cook for another 1-2 minutes.
4. Stir in the mushrooms and cook for 5 minutes.
5. Pour in the vegetable broth, dried thyme, and ground black pepper. Bring to a boil.
6. Reduce heat and simmer for 20-25 minutes, until the mushrooms are tender.
7. Stir in the skim milk and heat through without boiling.
8. Serve warm, garnished with fresh chives if desired.

Nutrition Info per Serving:
- Calories: 180
- Protein: 6g
- Carbohydrates: 22g
- Dietary Fiber: 4g
- Sugars: 8g
- Fat: 8g
- Saturated Fat: 1.5g
- Sodium: 170mg

Servings: 4
Cooking Time: 30 minutes

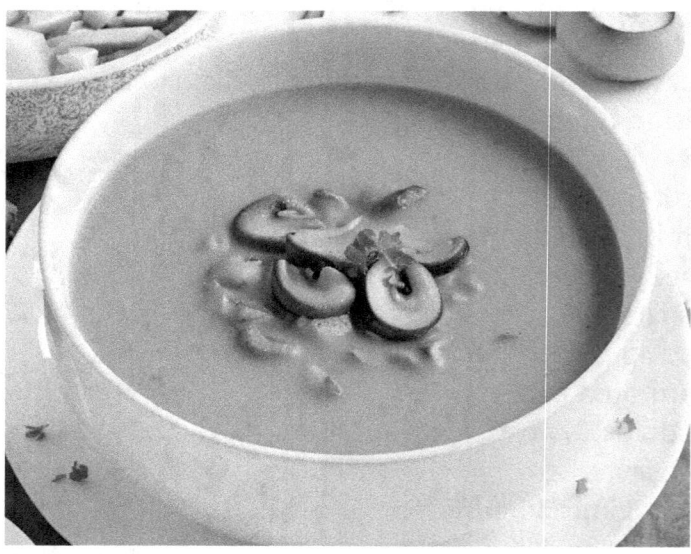

11. Zucchini and Basil Soup

Ingredients:
- 1 tbsp olive oil
- 1 onion, chopped
- 2 cloves garlic, minced
- 4 cups zucchini, chopped
- 4 cups low-sodium vegetable broth
- 1/2 tsp ground black pepper
- 1/2 cup fresh basil leaves
- 1/4 cup plain Greek yogurt (optional for garnish)

Instructions:
1. Heat the olive oil in a large pot over medium heat.
2. Add the onion and cook until softened, about 3-4 minutes.
3. Add the garlic and cook for another 1-2 minutes.
4. Stir in the chopped zucchini and cook for 5 minutes.
5. Pour in the vegetable broth and ground black pepper. Bring to a boil.
6. Reduce heat and simmer for 15-20 minutes, until the zucchini is tender.
7. Use an immersion blender to puree the soup until smooth (or transfer to a blender in batches).
8. Stir in the fresh basil leaves and cook for another 1-2 minutes.
9. Serve warm, garnished with a dollop of Greek yogurt if desired.

Nutrition Info per Serving:
- Calories: 140
- Protein: 4g
- Carbohydrates: 18g
- Dietary Fiber: 4g
- Sugars: 10g
- Fat: 6g
- Saturated Fat: 1g
- Sodium: 150mg

Servings: 4
Cooking Time: 30 minutes

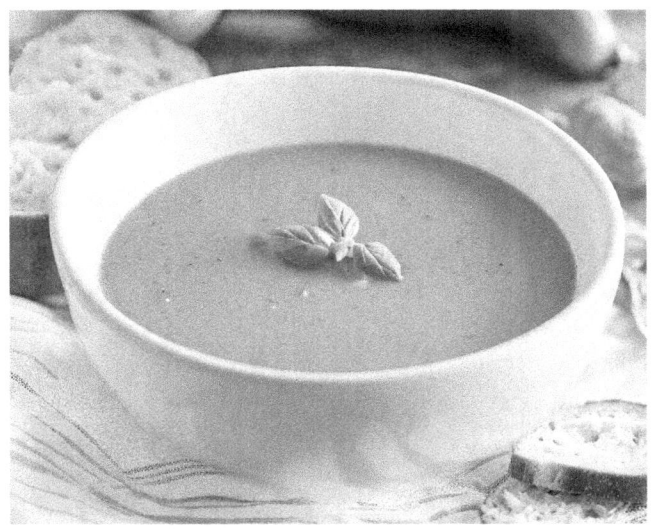

12. White Bean and Kale Soup

Ingredients:
- 1 tbsp olive oil
- 1 onion, chopped
- 2 cloves garlic, minced
- 1 carrot, chopped
- 1 celery stalk, chopped
- 1 can (15 oz) white beans, drained and rinsed
- 4 cups low-sodium vegetable broth
- 1/2 tsp dried thyme
- 1/2 tsp ground black pepper
- 4 cups kale, chopped

Instructions:
1. Heat the olive oil in a large pot over medium heat.
2. Add the onion and cook until softened, about 3-4 minutes.
3. Add the garlic and cook for another 1-2 minutes.
4. Stir in the carrot and celery, and cook for 5 minutes.
5. Pour in the vegetable broth, white beans, dried thyme, and ground black pepper. Bring to a boil.
6. Reduce heat and simmer for 20 minutes.
7. Stir in the chopped kale and cook for another 5 minutes, until wilted.
8. Serve warm.

Nutrition Info per Serving:
- Calories: 200
- Protein: 8g
- Carbohydrates: 30g
- Dietary Fiber: 10g
- Sugars: 5g
- Fat: 5g
- Saturated Fat: 1g
- Sodium: 180mg

Servings: 4
Cooking Time: 30 minutes

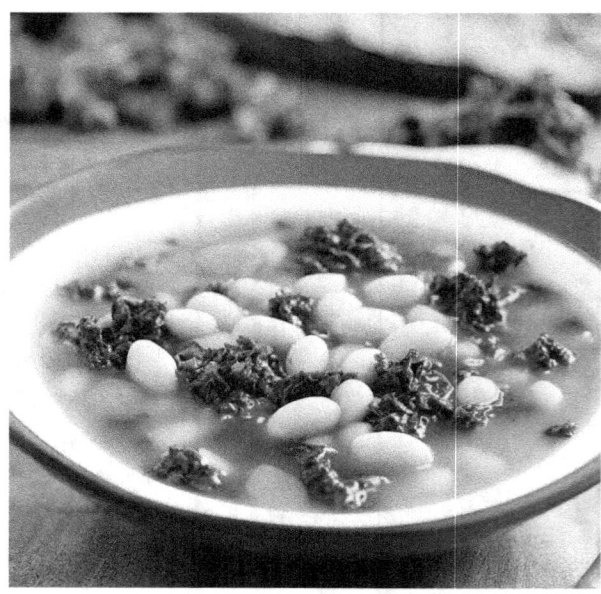

13. Black Bean Soup

Ingredients:
- 1 tbsp olive oil
- 1 onion, chopped
- 2 cloves garlic, minced
- 1 carrot, chopped
- 1 red bell pepper, chopped
- 2 cans (15 oz each) black beans, drained and rinsed
- 4 cups low-sodium vegetable broth
- 1 tsp ground cumin
- 1/2 tsp ground black pepper
- 1/4 cup fresh cilantro, chopped (optional for garnish)

Instructions:
1. Heat the olive oil in a large pot over medium heat.
2. Add the onion and cook until softened, about 3-4 minutes.
3. Add the garlic and cook for another 1-2 minutes.
4. Stir in the carrot and red bell pepper, and cook for 5 minutes.
5. Pour in the vegetable broth, black beans, ground cumin, and ground black pepper. Bring to a boil.
6. Reduce heat and simmer for 25-30 minutes, until the vegetables are tender.
7. Use an immersion blender to partially puree the soup, leaving some chunks for texture (or transfer half to a blender and puree, then return to the pot).
8. Serve warm, garnished with fresh cilantro if desired.

Nutrition Info per Serving:
- Calories: 220
- Protein: 10g
- Carbohydrates: 40g
- Dietary Fiber: 12g
- Sugars: 6g
- Fat: 5g
- Saturated Fat: 1g
- Sodium: 200mg

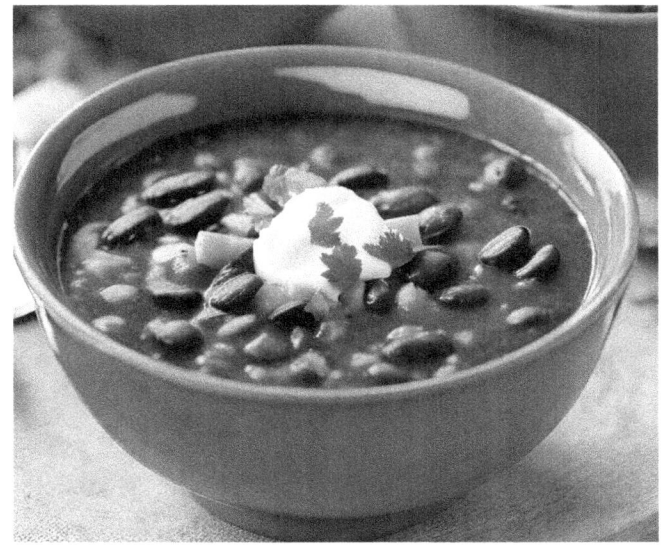

Servings: 4
Cooking Time: 35 minutes

14. Broccoli and Potato Soup

Ingredients:
- 1 tbsp olive oil
- 1 onion, chopped
- 2 cloves garlic, minced
- 2 large potatoes, peeled and chopped
- 4 cups broccoli florets
- 4 cups low-sodium vegetable broth
- 1/2 tsp ground black pepper
- 1/2 cup skim milk (or dairy-free alternative)
- 1/4 cup fresh chives, chopped (optional for garnish)

Instructions:
1. Heat the olive oil in a large pot over medium heat.
2. Add the onion and cook until softened, about 3-4 minutes.
3. Add the garlic and cook for another 1-2 minutes.
4. Stir in the potatoes and cook for 5 minutes.
5. Pour in the vegetable broth and ground black pepper. Bring to a boil.
6. Reduce heat and simmer for 15 minutes.
7. Add the broccoli florets and cook for another 10-15 minutes, until the vegetables are tender.
8. Use an immersion blender to puree the soup until smooth (or transfer to a blender in batches).
9. Stir in the skim milk and heat through without boiling.
10. Serve warm, garnished with fresh chives if desired.

Nutrition Info per Serving:
- Calories: 180
- Protein: 6g
- Carbohydrates: 28g
- Dietary Fiber: 6g
- Sugars: 4g
- Fat: 5g
- Saturated Fat: 1g
- Sodium: 160mg

Servings: 4
Cooking Time: 30 minutes

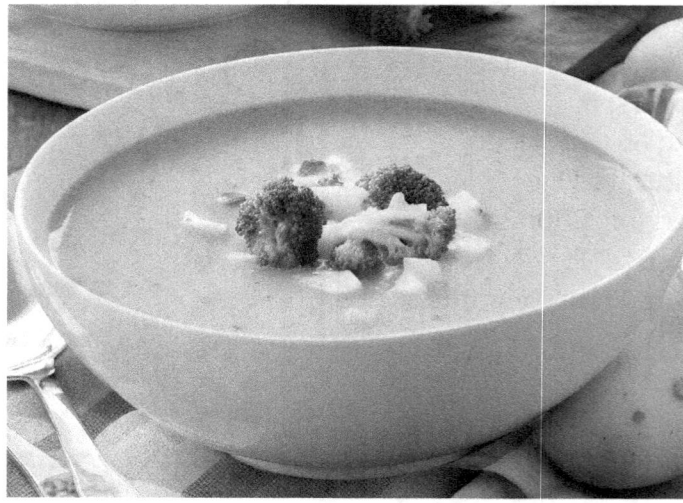

15. Turmeric and Cauliflower Soup

Ingredients:
- 1 tbsp olive oil
- 1 onion, chopped
- 2 cloves garlic, minced
- 1 head cauliflower, chopped
- 4 cups low-sodium vegetable broth
- 1 tsp ground turmeric
- 1/2 tsp ground black pepper
- 1/2 cup coconut milk
- 1/4 cup fresh cilantro, chopped (optional for garnish)

Instructions:
1. Heat the olive oil in a large pot over medium heat.
2. Add the onion and cook until softened, about 3-4 minutes.
3. Add the garlic and cook for another 1-2 minutes.
4. Stir in the chopped cauliflower and cook for 5 minutes.
5. Pour in the vegetable broth, ground turmeric, and ground black pepper. Bring to a boil.
6. Reduce heat and simmer for 20-25 minutes, until the cauliflower is tender.
7. Use an immersion blender to puree the soup until smooth (or transfer to a blender in batches).
8. Stir in the coconut milk and heat through without boiling.
9. Serve warm, garnished with fresh cilantro if desired.

Nutrition Info per Serving:
- Calories: 190
- Protein: 4g
- Carbohydrates: 16g
- Dietary Fiber: 6g
- Sugars: 4g
- Fat: 12g
- Saturated Fat: 5g
- Sodium: 150mg

Servings: 4
Cooking Time: 30 minutes

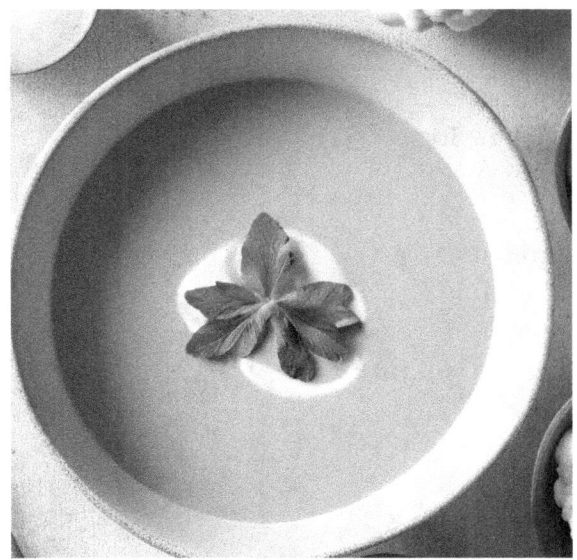

16. Italian Vegetable Stew

Ingredients:
- 1 tbsp olive oil
- 1 onion, chopped
- 2 cloves garlic, minced
- 2 carrots, chopped
- 2 celery stalks, chopped
- 1 zucchini, chopped
- 1 can (14.5 oz) diced tomatoes, no salt added
- 4 cups low-sodium vegetable broth
- 1 can (15 oz) cannellini beans, drained and rinsed
- 1 tsp dried oregano
- 1/2 tsp ground black pepper
- 1/4 cup fresh basil, chopped (optional for garnish)

Instructions:
1. Heat the olive oil in a large pot over medium heat.
2. Add the onion and cook until softened, about 3-4 minutes.
3. Add the garlic and cook for another 1-2 minutes.
4. Stir in the carrots, celery, and zucchini. Cook for 5 minutes.
5. Pour in the diced tomatoes, vegetable broth, and beans. Bring to a boil.
6. Stir in the dried oregano and ground black pepper.
7. Reduce heat and simmer for 25-30 minutes, until the vegetables are tender.
8. Serve warm, garnished with fresh basil if desired.

Nutrition Info per Serving:
- Calories: 220
- Protein: 8g
- Carbohydrates: 35g
- Dietary Fiber: 10g
- Sugars: 8g
- Fat: 5g
- Saturated Fat: 0.5g
- Sodium: 180mg

Servings: 4
Cooking Time: 35 minutes

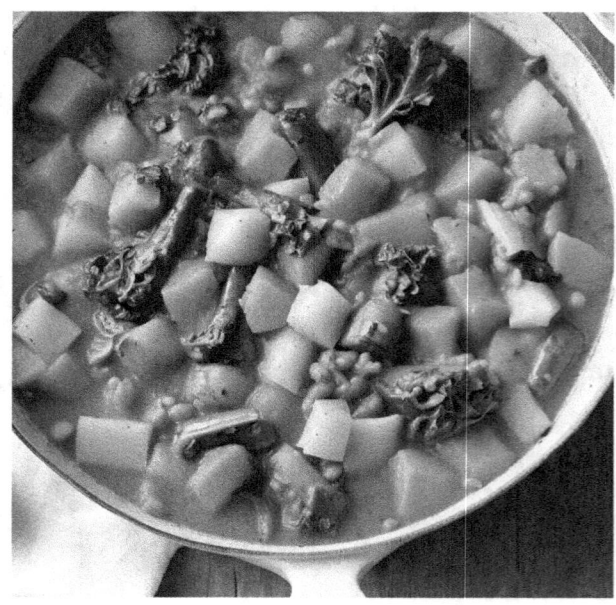

17. Potato and Green Bean Soup

Ingredients:
- 1 tbsp olive oil
- 1 onion, chopped
- 2 cloves garlic, minced
- 4 potatoes, peeled and chopped
- 2 cups green beans, trimmed and cut into 1-inch pieces
- 4 cups low-sodium vegetable broth
- 1/2 tsp ground black pepper
- 1/4 cup fresh dill, chopped (optional for garnish)

Instructions:
1. Heat the olive oil in a large pot over medium heat.
2. Add the onion and cook until softened, about 3-4 minutes.
3. Add the garlic and cook for another 1-2 minutes.
4. Stir in the potatoes and cook for 5 minutes.
5. Pour in the vegetable broth and ground black pepper. Bring to a boil.
6. Reduce heat and simmer for 15-20 minutes, until the potatoes are tender.
7. Add the green beans and cook for another 5-7 minutes, until tender.
8. Serve warm, garnished with fresh dill if desired.

Nutrition Info per Serving:
- Calories: 180
- Protein: 5g
- Carbohydrates: 32g
- Dietary Fiber: 6g
- Sugars: 4g
- Fat: 4g
- Saturated Fat: 0.5g
- Sodium: 160mg

Servings: 4
Cooking Time: 30 minutes

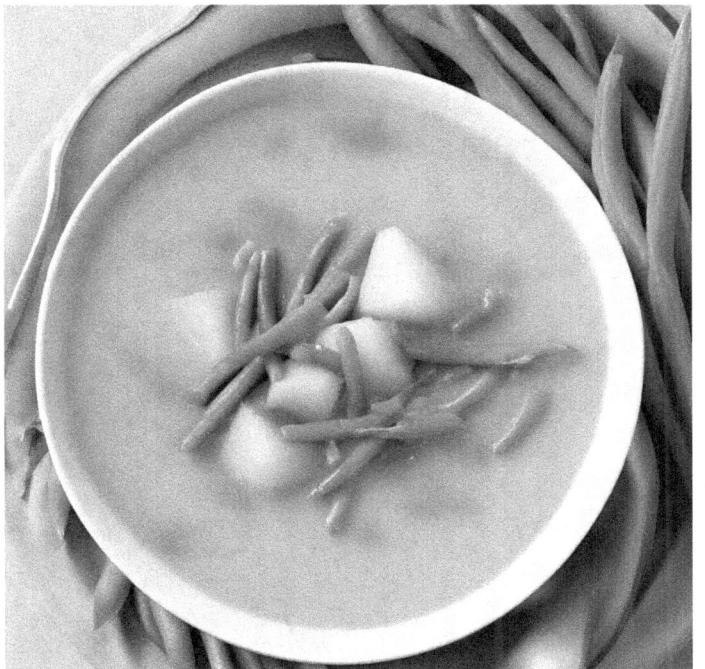

18. Chard and White Bean Soup

Ingredients:
- 1 tbsp olive oil
- 1 onion, chopped
- 2 cloves garlic, minced
- 4 cups chard, chopped
- 1 can (15 oz) white beans, drained and rinsed
- 4 cups low-sodium vegetable broth
- 1/2 tsp ground black pepper
- 1/4 cup fresh parsley, chopped (optional for garnish)

Instructions:
1. Heat the olive oil in a large pot over medium heat.
2. Add the onion and cook until softened, about 3-4 minutes.
3. Add the garlic and cook for another 1-2 minutes.
4. Stir in the chard and cook for 5 minutes.
5. Pour in the vegetable broth, white beans, and ground black pepper. Bring to a boil.
6. Reduce heat and simmer for 15-20 minutes, until the chard is tender.
7. Serve warm, garnished with fresh parsley if desired.

Nutrition Info per Serving:
- Calories: 180
- Protein: 8g
- Carbohydrates: 30g
- Dietary Fiber: 8g
- Sugars: 4g
- Fat: 4g
- Saturated Fat: 0.5g
- Sodium: 160mg

Servings: 4
Cooking Time: 25 minutes

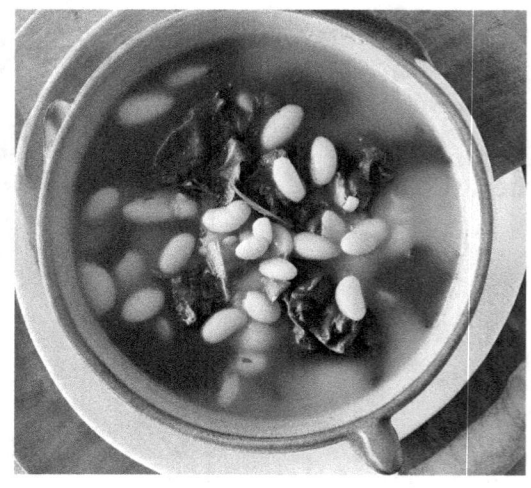

8-WEEK MEAL PLAN

Week 1
Monday:
- Breakfast: Banana Oatmeal Porridge
- Lunch: Chicken and Spinach Stew
- Dinner: Grilled Salmon with Dill
- Snack: Carrot and Ginger Juice

Tuesday:
- Breakfast: Smoothie Bowl
- Lunch: Lentil and Spinach Soup
- Dinner: Poached Cod
- Snack: Papaya Salad

Wednesday:
- Breakfast: Egg White Scramble
- Lunch: Chickpea and Vegetable Stew
- Dinner: Baked Tilapia with Lemon Pepper
- Snack: Oat Bran Muffins

Thursday:
- Breakfast: Avocado Toast on Whole Grain Bread
- Lunch: Split Pea Soup
- Dinner: Shrimp and Vegetable Stir-Fry
- Snack: Buckwheat Pancakes

Friday:
- Breakfast: Peaches and Cream Smoothie
- Lunch: Pumpkin Soup
- Dinner: Steamed Mussels with Garlic and Herbs
- Snack: Vegetable Soup

Saturday:
- Breakfast: Carrot and Ginger Juice
- Lunch: Turkey and Sweet Potato Skillet
- Dinner: Sole Meunière
- Snack: Chia Seed Pudding

Sunday:
- Breakfast: Cucumber Tomato Sandwich
- Lunch: Broccoli and Potato Soup
- Dinner: Stuffed Squid with Herbed Rice
- Snack: Berry Fruit Salad

Week 2

Monday:
- Breakfast: Barley Porridge
- Lunch: Pea and Mint Soup
- Dinner: Herb-Roasted Turkey Breast
- Snack: Pumpkin Soup

Tuesday:
- Breakfast: Smoothie Bowl
- Lunch: Red Lentil and Carrot Stew
- Dinner: Chicken and Mushroom Casserole
- Snack: Papaya Salad

Wednesday:
- Breakfast: Egg White Scramble
- Lunch: Vegetable Minestrone
- Dinner: Grilled Shrimp Skewers
- Snack: Oat Bran Muffins

Thursday:
- Breakfast: Avocado Toast on Whole Grain Bread
- Lunch: White Bean and Kale Soup
- Dinner: Baked Trout with Rosemary
- Snack: Buckwheat Pancakes

Friday:
- Breakfast: Peaches and Cream Smoothie
- Lunch: Vegetable and Chickpea Stew
- Dinner: Grilled Turkey and Pineapple
- Snack: Vegetable Soup

Saturday:
- Breakfast: Carrot and Ginger Juice
- Lunch: Sweet Potato and Lentil Soup
- Dinner: Chicken Pepperoni Marinara
- Snack: Chia Seed Pudding

Sunday:
- Breakfast: Cucumber Tomato Sandwich
- Lunch: Beet and Ginger Soup
- Dinner: Chicken Ratatouille
- Snack: Berry Fruit Salad

Week 3

Monday:
- Breakfast: Barley Porridge
- Lunch: Potato and Green Bean Soup
- Dinner: Turkey and Rice Pilaf
- Snack: Pumpkin Soup

Tuesday:
- Breakfast: Smoothie Bowl
- Lunch: Corn and Potato Chowder
- Dinner: Broiled Scallops with Paprika
- Snack: Papaya Salad

Wednesday:
- Breakfast: Egg White Scramble
- Lunch: Chard and White Bean Soup
- Dinner: Grilled Eel with Teriyaki Sauce
- Snack: Oat Bran Muffins

Thursday:
- Breakfast: Avocado Toast on Whole Grain Bread
- Lunch: Italian Vegetable Stew
- Dinner: Chicken Piccata
- Snack: Buckwheat Pancakes

Friday:
- Breakfast: Peaches and Cream Smoothie
- Lunch: Turmeric and Cauliflower Soup
- Dinner: Marinated Anchovies with Garlic and Vinegar
- Snack: Vegetable Soup

Saturday:
- Breakfast: Carrot and Ginger Juice
- Lunch: Broccoli and Potato Soup
- Dinner: Balsamic Chicken
- Snack: Chia Seed Pudding

Sunday:
- Breakfast: Cucumber Tomato Sandwich
- Lunch: Miso Soup with Tofu and Seaweed
- Dinner: Turkey Quinoa Stuffed Peppers
- Snack: Berry Fruit Salad

Week 4

Monday:
- Breakfast: Barley Porridge
- Lunch: Zucchini and Basil Soup
- Dinner: Seared Tuna with Sesame Seeds
- Snack: Pumpkin Soup

Tuesday:
- Breakfast: Smoothie Bowl
- Lunch: Black Bean Soup
- Dinner: Poached Chicken Salad
- Snack: Papaya Salad

Wednesday:
- Breakfast: Egg White Scramble
- Lunch: Sweet Potato and Lentil Soup
- Dinner: Grilled Shrimp Skewers
- Snack: Oat Bran Muffins

Thursday:
- Breakfast: Avocado Toast on Whole Grain Bread
- Lunch: White Bean and Kale Soup
- Dinner: Lemon Garlic Chicken
- Snack: Buckwheat Pancakes

Friday:
- Breakfast: Peaches and Cream Smoothie
- Lunch: Vegetable and Chickpea Stew
- Dinner: Grilled Turkey and Pineapple
- Snack: Vegetable Soup

Saturday:
- Breakfast: Carrot and Ginger Juice
- Lunch: Red Lentil and Carrot Stew
- Dinner: Chicken and Broccoli Alfredo
- Snack: Chia Seed Pudding

Sunday:
- Breakfast: Cucumber Tomato Sandwich
- Lunch: Beet and Ginger Soup
- Dinner: Monkfish with Saffron Broth
- Snack: Berry Fruit Salad

Week 5

Monday:
- Breakfast: Mango Smoothie
- Lunch: Bean and Barley Soup
- Dinner: Turkey Meatballs
- Snack: Sautéed Vegetables

Tuesday:
- Breakfast: Spelt Toast with Banana
- Lunch: Cabbage Soup
- Dinner: Smoked Turkey Wrap
- Snack: Almond Milk Porridge

Wednesday:
- Breakfast: Boiled Potatoes with Dill
- Lunch: Miso Soup with Tofu and Seaweed
- Dinner: Chicken Congee
- Snack: Vegetable Omelette

Thursday:
- Breakfast: Papaya Salad
- Lunch: Broccoli and Potato Soup
- Dinner: Poached Cod
- Snack: Berry Fruit Salad

Friday:
- Breakfast: Peaches and Cream Smoothie
- Lunch: Black Bean Soup
- Dinner: Grilled Shrimp Skewers
- Snack: Buckwheat Pancakes

Saturday:
- Breakfast: Smoothie Bowl
- Lunch: Red Lentil and Carrot Stew
- Dinner: Chicken and Mushroom Casserole
- Snack: Vegetable Soup

Sunday:
- Breakfast: Cucumber Tomato Sandwich
- Lunch: Zucchini and Basil Soup
- Dinner: Balsamic Chicken
- Snack: Chia Seed Pudding

Week 6

Monday:
- Breakfast: Barley Porridge
- Lunch: White Bean and Kale Soup
- Dinner: Lemon Garlic Chicken
- Snack: Vegetable Soup

Tuesday:
- Breakfast: Smoothie Bowl
- Lunch: Italian Vegetable Stew
- Dinner: Marinated Anchovies with Garlic and Vinegar
- Snack: Papaya Salad

Wednesday:
- Breakfast: Egg White Scramble
- Lunch: Potato and Green Bean Soup
- Dinner: Grilled Turkey and Pineapple
- Snack: Oat Bran Muffins

Thursday:
- Breakfast: Avocado Toast on Whole Grain Bread
- Lunch: Corn and Potato Chowder
- Dinner: Grilled Eel with Teriyaki Sauce
- Snack: Buckwheat Pancakes

Friday:
- Breakfast: Peaches and Cream Smoothie
- Lunch: Chard and White Bean Soup
- Dinner: Chicken Piccata
- Snack: Vegetable Soup

Saturday:
- Breakfast: Carrot and Ginger Juice
- Lunch: Broccoli and Potato Soup
- Dinner: Poached Chicken Salad
- Snack: Chia Seed Pudding

Sunday:
- Breakfast: Cucumber Tomato Sandwich
- Lunch: Sweet Potato and Lentil Soup
- Dinner: Chicken and Broccoli Alfredo
- Snack: Berry Fruit Salad

Week 7

Monday:
- Breakfast: Barley Porridge
- Lunch: Miso Soup with Tofu and Seaweed
- Dinner: Monkfish with Saffron Broth
- Snack: Pumpkin Soup

Tuesday:
- Breakfast: Smoothie Bowl
- Lunch: Beet and Ginger Soup
- Dinner: Seared Tuna with Sesame Seeds
- Snack: Papaya Salad

Wednesday:
- Breakfast: Egg White Scramble
- Lunch: Italian Vegetable Stew
- Dinner: Broiled Scallops with Paprika
- Snack: Oat Bran Muffins

Thursday:
- Breakfast: Avocado Toast on Whole Grain Bread
- Lunch: Potato and Green Bean Soup
- Dinner: Stuffed Squid with Herbed Rice
- Snack: Buckwheat Pancakes

Friday:
- Breakfast: Peaches and Cream Smoothie
- Lunch: Corn and Potato Chowder
- Dinner: Chicken Pepperoni Marinara
- Snack: Vegetable Soup

Saturday:
- Breakfast: Carrot and Ginger Juice
- Lunch: Zucchini and Basil Soup
- Dinner: Grilled Shrimp Skewers
- Snack: Chia Seed Pudding

Sunday:
- Breakfast: Cucumber Tomato Sandwich
- Lunch: White Bean and Kale Soup
- Dinner: Herb-Roasted Turkey Breast
- Snack: Berry Fruit Salad

Week 8

Monday:
- Breakfast: Barley Porridge
- Lunch: Red Lentil and Carrot Stew
- Dinner: Chicken Congee
- Snack: Vegetable Soup

Tuesday:
- Breakfast: Smoothie Bowl
- Lunch: Black Bean Soup
- Dinner: Balsamic Chicken
- Snack: Papaya Salad

Wednesday:
- Breakfast: Egg White Scramble
- Lunch: Chard and White Bean Soup
- Dinner: Marinated Anchovies with Garlic and Vinegar
- Snack: Oat Bran Muffins

Thursday:
- Breakfast: Avocado Toast on Whole Grain Bread
- Lunch: Sweet Potato and Lentil Soup
- Dinner: Poached Cod
- Snack: Buckwheat Pancakes

Friday:
- Breakfast: Peaches and Cream Smoothie
- Lunch: Potato and Green Bean Soup
- Dinner: Turkey and Rice Pilaf
- Snack: Vegetable Soup

Saturday:
- Breakfast: Carrot and Ginger Juice
- Lunch: Beet and Ginger Soup
- Dinner: Grilled Eel with Teriyaki Sauce
- Snack: Chia Seed Pudding

Sunday:
- Breakfast: Cucumber Tomato Sandwich
- Lunch: Zucchini and Basil Soup
- Dinner: Chicken and Mushroom Casserole
- Snack: Berry Fruit Salad

WEEKLY MEAL PLANNER + WORKBOOK

	BREAKFAST	LUNCH	DINNER	SNACKS
MONDAY				
TUESDAY				
WEDNESDAY				
THURSDAY				
FRIDAY				
SATURDAY				
SUNDAY				

What are your main goals for starting a pancreatitis-friendly diet?

....

....

....

....

....

....

WEEKLY MEAL PLANNER + WORKBOOK

	BREAKFAST	LUNCH	DINNER	SNACKS
MONDAY				
TUESDAY				
WEDNESDAY				
THURSDAY				
FRIDAY				
SATURDAY				
SUNDAY				

How do you currently feel about your understanding of pancreatitis and its dietary requirements?

....

....

....

....

....

....

WEEKLY MEAL PLANNER + WORKBOOK

	BREAKFAST	LUNCH	DINNER	SNACKS
MONDAY				
TUESDAY				
WEDNESDAY				
THURSDAY				
FRIDAY				
SATURDAY				
SUNDAY				

What challenges do you anticipate facing when changing your diet for pancreatitis?

....
....
....
....
....
....

WEEKLY MEAL PLANNER + WORKBOOK

	BREAKFAST	LUNCH	DINNER	SNACKS
MONDAY				
TUESDAY				
WEDNESDAY				
THURSDAY				
FRIDAY				
SATURDAY				
SUNDAY				

List three of your favorite meals or snacks. How might these be adapted to fit a pancreatitis-friendly diet?

....

....

....

....

....

....

WEEKLY MEAL PLANNER + WORKBOOK

	BREAKFAST	LUNCH	DINNER	SNACKS
MONDAY				
TUESDAY				
WEDNESDAY				
THURSDAY				
FRIDAY				
SATURDAY				
SUNDAY				

Which recipes from the cookbook are you most excited to try first, and why?

....

....

....

....

....

....

WEEKLY MEAL PLANNER + WORKBOOK

	BREAKFAST	LUNCH	DINNER	SNACKS
MONDAY				
TUESDAY				
WEDNESDAY				
THURSDAY				
FRIDAY				
SATURDAY				
SUNDAY				

What cooking methods (e.g., grilling, baking, steaming) do you find most appealing for preparing pancreatitis-friendly meals?

....

....

....

....

....

....

WEEKLY MEAL PLANNER + WORKBOOK

	BREAKFAST	LUNCH	DINNER	SNACKS
MONDAY				
TUESDAY				
WEDNESDAY				
THURSDAY				
FRIDAY				
SATURDAY				
SUNDAY				

What pantry staples and fresh ingredients will you need to stock up on to follow the recipes in this cookbook?

....

....

....

....

....

....

WEEKLY MEAL PLANNER + WORKBOOK

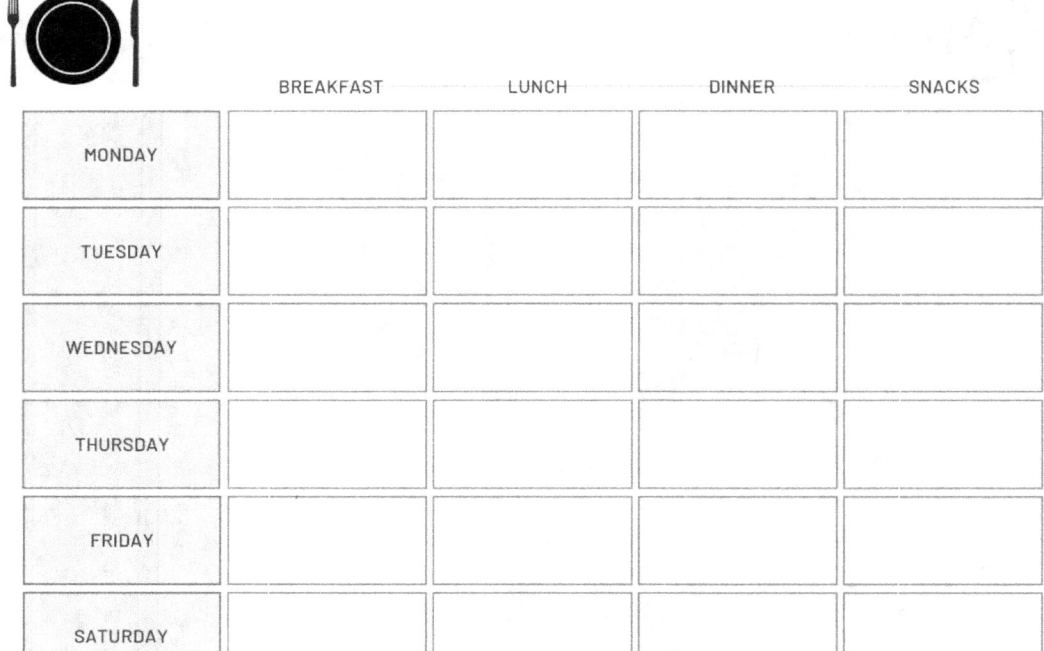

How will you ensure you stay hydrated throughout the day? List two strategies.

....

....

....

....

....

WEEKLY MEAL PLANNER + WORKBOOK

	BREAKFAST	LUNCH	DINNER	SNACKS
MONDAY				
TUESDAY				
WEDNESDAY				
THURSDAY				
FRIDAY				
SATURDAY				
SUNDAY				

How will you handle dining out or eating at social gatherings while maintaining your pancreatitis-friendly diet?

....

....

....

....

....

....

WEEKLY MEAL PLANNER + WORKBOOK

	BREAKFAST	LUNCH	DINNER	SNACKS
MONDAY				
TUESDAY				
WEDNESDAY				
THURSDAY				
FRIDAY				
SATURDAY				
SUNDAY				

List three breakfast recipes from the cookbook that you want to try. How do they fit into your morning routine?

....

....

....

....

....

WEEKLY MEAL PLANNER + WORKBOOK

	BREAKFAST	LUNCH	DINNER	SNACKS
MONDAY				
TUESDAY				
WEDNESDAY				
THURSDAY				
FRIDAY				
SATURDAY				
SUNDAY				

How do you plan to handle cravings for foods that are not pancreatitis-friendly?

....

....

....

....

....

....

Scan the QR code below to get a surprise bonus!

www.ingramcontent.com/pod-product-compliance
Lightning Source LLC
Chambersburg PA
CBHW082204220526
45470CB00010B/3048